THE POWER TO NAVIGATE LIFE

Your Journey to Freedom

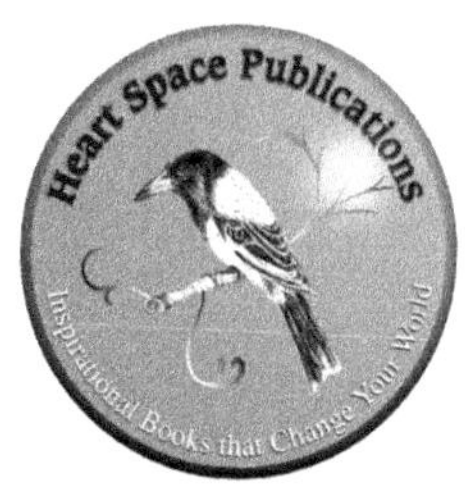

Publisthed by
Heart Space Publications
PO Box 1085
Daylesford
Victoria
34660
Australia

Tel +61 450263348
www.heartspacebooks.com
pat@heartspacebooks.com

Designed by **timson**.co | www.timson.co

ISBN 978-0-9924338-0-2

To learn more about Tony Fahkry's work, go to:

www.tonyfahkry.com

TONY FAHKRY

Holistic Health & Self-Empowerment
Presenter | Author

Founder of *The Power to Navigate Life,* Tony is a leading holistic, health and self-empowerment specialist. He brings over ten years' experience at the highest level as a health professional, corporate and public speaker, author and coach. His understanding and integration of mind and body concepts bridges the gap between health, well-being and human behavior

Tony's *The Power to Navigate Life* program, has presented to corporate companies across Australia. The program teaches participants how to achieve continued mental, emotional and physical well-being using his easy to follow principles. This book contains the principles espoused in the program.

Tony has worked with Bupa Australia presenting The Power to Navigate Life seminars in Melbourne and Sydney to Ericsson employees. Tony is a regular monthly contributor to Bupa's online magazine, BeWell. He has published articles for UltraFit magazine and has completed an eight week mental resilience, health and wellbeing program for the Coles senior executive team.

He is a regular contributor (over one hundred articles) for online EzineArticles.com, as well as for ArticleBase.com on personal growth, empowerment, inspiration, health and well-being, mind and body matters, and self-awareness.

Tony is also the head of Core Conditioning for Triathlon Victoria's coaching program, which he presents quarterly. He currently works with a number of Australia's leading CEO's and corporate executives.

He has written two eBooks on health and wellbeing and self-development. These are available to download via his website.

FOREWORD

by Eldon Taylor, PhD, FAPA

You are about to embark on a journey that will enhance your life and immerse you in the essences of your quintessential being.

The *Power to Navigate Life* offers concepts that will connect deeply within your being and consequently raise a new awareness of your potential. You will come to understand, not just intellectually, but also at a deeper emotional level, that, there are no mistakes in life—only outcomes, and that you are in charge of those outcomes.

In The Power to Navigate Life, Tony discusses his own life lessons and challenges including his life threatening bout with cancer, distilling his insight through the lens of universal rules. Using these rules, he teaches us how to welcome each new challenge as an opportunity, just as we might welcome news of something like a pay raise. In his words, "Saying YES means embracing the essence of the experience that is before us."

There is warmth in Tony's words, that seems to reach in and somehow touch our souls and although we already know deep down everything he teaches, we have failed to remember them. I particularly like the way Tony removes any judgment and notion of failure from his approach. One of his lessons had great appeal to me, because it described some of my own personal experiences. Again in his words, "Sometimes in life the wrong turn can and will deliver us to the right place in time."

In the end, this is a journey that will reveal self-sabotaging and self-destructive patterns, while emphasizing the liberation that comes from not just realizing you have the power to create your own reality, but from learning how to do so from this point on.

A good self-help book should produce an experience, deliver the motivation necessary for you to follow through, and leave you with a new level of confidence with which to continue your journey. The Power to Navigate Life does precisely this. I highly recommend the book and I know that you will appreciate and prosper as a result of your experience with it.

Enjoy your read

Eldon Taylor, PhD, FAPA

NY Times Bestselling Author of Choices and Illusions

Testimonials

Tony Fahkry lets us see into his soul, forged in near-tragedy, but resulting in a layered stream of consciousness, shared with us in this book. Tony's goal is not to embed us in his life, but rather in the growth of his person and personality as he navigated the twists and turns of his soul's response to all life bought. Thus we as readers are immersed in his words and his enlightenment, so saving us the journey he embarked on and successfully completed – as if a travel book for the spirit, Tony's brave and compelling insights lead us to contemplate our own approach to adversity and the freedom that results if we try

Roy Sugarman PhD
Clinical Psychologist, Neuropsychologist and Author of Saving your life one day at a time and Motivation for coaches & personal trainers.

Tony Fahkry provides a blueprint for well-being that should be read by anybody who wants a healthy life. He shows convincingly the importance of a positive state of mind for good physical health. More than that, good emotional health is vital. Life is too short not to heed the lessons of this book.

Jerome Fahrer
Director ACIL Allen Consulting

Most of us know what we have to do to be healthy but battle to overcome the negative chatter inside our heads that sabotages our efforts. Despite much effort the "chatter" inevitably wins the day and we end up back where we started. There is no easy path to fitness and good health; it requires effort and discipline to get there and effort and discipline to stay fit and healthy. There are many books that set out the physical things that you have to do to achieve fitness and good health but there is a dearth of information about the hard part – the battle with the negative chatter that sabotages the best efforts. As my trainer Tony Fahkry gave me the mental tools necessary to overcome all the "negative" chatter that sabotaged my efforts to improve my health. In this book Tony has revealed his secrets about the mental tools that can set you on your path to good health.

Robert Hay
Property Law Barrister. Victorian Bar

CONTENTS

The Power to Navigate Life

You Never Know What Life Had Planned For You

Over a decade ago, *The Power to Navigate Life* began as my own personal journey. In fact, I recall that precise moment my life began to change. It was when I heard the rheumatologist utter the word CANCER and instantaneously my equilibrium was shattered. Life as I knew it would never be the same.

Immediately, the word death came to mind at the mention of cancer. Death and disease had become as familiar friends over the years (my father died from complications of type II diabetes), so I knew all too well their correlation.

But as time progressed, I came to understand the underlying mechanisms of the brain and began to appreciate the mind's desire to make associations. In actual fact, the words *death* and *cancer* were only related by association in a game played by the mind. I needed to begin to make new associations, because this was no longer a game—it was my life.

However, this book is not the story of my life nor is it about my battle to overcome cancer when the odds were stacked against me, as there are plenty of such stories lining the bookshelves. I prefer not to dwell on disease, because I do not feel as though I am its victim. Nor have I ever wanted illness to be a focal point or defining element of who I am or the message I am here to communicate. Because the result of my cancer was, in fact, the greatest gift imaginable—**an awakening to realization of the perfection of life**. So my journey with cancer became a story about how to embrace life, irrespective of background, education, health challenges or otherwise.

You may wonder how exactly I awoke to realize life's perfection. The transformation itself was not a singular, instantaneous moment in which I awoke fully enlightened. Rather, it was **a natural unfolding of energy that merged within my inner being**. In a sense, I had to get out of my own way; I needed to step back and simply allow the process to unfold, by allowing the energy to flow, instead of resisting what I thought I wanted my life to be.

Over time, these subtle changes or shifts to my outlook and thinking had a huge impact on my life. Yes, there were times when I had no idea what was happening to me and sometimes I still do not fully understand what comes next. Yet, within me exists an *inner knowing* that everything will be ok, as though I am being guided. As long as I keep taking the necessary steps, I know that I will be supported.

Since the time of my cancer and subsequent awakening, I have come in contact with many people who have endured similar health scares. Few of them, have had such a life-altering wake up. Certainly, they are all grateful to be alive, capable of living life to the fullest. However, surviving cancer does not automatically make one aware of how fortunate they are to be alive. Instead of living vibrantly in the perfection of life, many return to the safety of their old beliefs, grateful only for having escaped death.

But living fully consists of more than knowing how to escape death. Life in its fullest sense reveals itself through you, as an expression of energy. If you allow life to move through you, you can **become the expression of life's energy**. When you resist this energy, you end up blocking a life that is unfolding specifically for you. Utilizing this mindset, no situation is ever as bad as you imagine or expect it to be. Participating fully in life requires only three simple ingredients: **time, patience, and trust**.

Within this book, I will discuss two concepts, drawing upon analogies of the different ways of living life. By the close of this book, you will come to understand that there are no mistakes in life—only outcomes. You will discover a force—an expression of life—that is exhilarating and deeply profound. You will also be instructed about how to work with universal forces and use them to guide your life. When you live by the Universe's rules, life begins to serve *you*. It serves you because *you are the expression of life itself.*

Far too many people discount the extraordinary messages that are contained within their own life story. These unique messages that appear through life are often opportunities disguised as challenges. These challenges allow us to become more than we are--more than we believe possible. We can only become more than we are by saying *YES* to life. Saying *YES* means embracing the essence of the experience that is before us. **Ultimately, it means showing less resistance to the circumstances that arise within each moment.**

The Power to Navigate Life is a book about realizing that there is more to life than what we have been told. More to life than paying bills, working at a job that we dislike or being in a relationship that does not serve us.

The Power to Navigate Life is a way of life centered on human potential. This potential stirs within each of us and can only be awakened when we dare to examine our deepest selves. For **within the deepest self lies an emptiness waiting to be filled with miracles.** This only happens if we are willing to get out of our own way and allow the process to unfold.

In creating *The Power to Navigate Life*, my aim and purpose was to teach participants how to view life from a different perspective. To illustrate how we continually create the circumstances of our life through childhood programs. These programs are beliefs, thoughts, ideas or anything else that we may have picked up from our environment, which allows us to create a perception or an image of our world.

The truth of the matter is that you are far more than your beliefs, thoughts or anything else you deemed possible for yourself. In order to awaken to a new reality and see life from a different perspective, it is essential that you look at life through a new lens. Your new way of seeing can only transpire when you abolish the old paradigms and the old way of thinking in order to pave a way for the fresh, new and vital energy that can permeate through your mind and body. **You have the power to create your reality from this moment onwards.**

While reading this book, I invite you to put away any preconceived ideas of what you have learned about life. Put away any mental constructs of what life has delivered so far; for in doing so, you might believe that you have been unfairly treated, taken advantage of, or even wronged.

You may have also formed beliefs about what reality is. However, this is *your* reality: *your* version, shaped by *your* perceptions, values and beliefs. I am here to show you a different reality.

For instance, if you continue to attract the wrong type of intimate relationships, being aware that you are creating these circumstances allows you to attract harmonious intimacy, instead of failed relationships. Power is earned through your willingness to shift your awareness.

And what if your problems led you to discover a new ways of approaching your difficulties? What I am suggesting is that **sometimes in life the wrong turn can and will deliver us to the right place and time.** Luckily, the right place is **HERE** and the right time is **NOW**!

If your reality, your world, is lived in such a way that you are dissatisfied and your senses are muted, you may continually be up against obstacles, dead-ends, rejections, failures and many other unwelcome surprises that arise along the way.

But there are good surprises, too, and you have picked up this book for a reason. Whether it was given to you by another person or you discovered it in your search for answers to life's persistent questions, this book is intended to guide you on your journey. Along the way, I hope you discover insights that might challenge all you have come to believe about life.

The Power to Navigate Life is a program like no other. It is the culmination of over ten years of personal experience, as well as the observations working one-on-one with clients and facilitating workshops and seminars.

The Power to Navigate Life offers an opportunity to step into a new way of creating your reality. As you read and study this book, try the principles and adapt them into your life. Observe the changes within your own life, for these changes are an indication of changing awareness. When your level of awareness begins to evolve and change, so will your level of consciousness begin to adapt and evolve.

 This higher state of human development advances our consciousness level from a primitive mind to higher states and a more evolved mind-set. Do not be discouraged if you find yourself relapsing from time to time. This is a normal part of the process as your mind begins to expand, creating new horizons from which to create your future.

It is my desire for you to fully embrace the principles of this program. The chapters have been organised in such a way so as to guide you through the program. I suggest you first read through the book and then return back to the chapters that you found difficult to digest.

I wish you great health and happiness in your life and trust from this point forward that you will be begin to create a new perspective from which to experience life. *The Power to Navigate Life* is an invitation to live that experience.

Tony FAHKRY

CHAPTER ONE

Parked versus Navigate Life

The Principles of Navigating Life

"The doctor of the future will give no medicine, but will interest her or his patients in the care of the human frame, in a proper diet and in the cause and prevention of disease."

Thomas Edison

There are three main principles underlying *The Power to Navigate Life: Health & Well-being, Personal Power* and *Health & Vibrant Life.* The first, *Health & Well-being,* is the springboard from which a prosperous life can emerge.

It has almost become a mainstay in society that the human body will inevitably break down. I do not think Mother Nature is so cruel as that to impose such limitations upon us. If we look back to our childhood, most can clearly see that a large portion of our early life was lived with a higher degree of health and well-being.

As we transition into our teenage years and adult life, we begin adopting practices that are subsequently detrimental to our long-term health – even though our bodies still manage to maintain a certain level of health. Yet despite this, people continually suppress Mother Nature's drive to optimise their well-being through inappropriate nutrition, recreational drugs, stress, and other lifestyle habits.

It takes some decades for the human body to manifest illness and disease.

In many cases it is not brought on suddenly, despite what people think when they learn of someone who experiences a heart attack. In these instance there may have been years of neglect with poor nutrition and inadequate lifestyle choices.

The Power to Navigate Life offers you an opportunity to experience an abundant, rich and prosperous life by developing sound health and well-being habits from this point forward. *The Power to Navigate Life* roadmap begins with health and well-being for this is the foundation that will carry your body over the coming decades.

During my time working one-on-one with clients, I consulted with many professional corporate executives who were close to retirement. Many of these people had accumulated a retirement plan that would see them well into their later years. Unfortunately, due to poor lifestyle choices during the early years, much of this retirement plan will be spent on medical bills, rather than enjoying their retirement. It is my wish that you do not get lulled into making the same choices.

Through awareness, you are able to choose more intelligently how you treat your body. In doing so, your body will offer you a level of health and well-being that will enable you to experience a rich and fulfilling life. It is no joy to have all the money in the world but lying in a hospital bed living with regret.

Your health and well-being are your higher states of wealth, for no person can ever deny you this. It is for you to choose each and every day how you treat and respect your body.

The second principle of *The Power to Navigate Life* roadmap is *Personal Power*. I believe that when we attain a higher state of health we create a level of *Personal Power* that enables us to create the ideal circumstances of our life. A higher state of health is one that offers the union of mind and body as one, rather than separate, as the Western model has espouses.

Recall for a moment people who in their later years suffered illness or disease. Note their lack of intensity toward life. They would have you know that they would pay any amount of money to reclaim their health.

Often it is too late to go back and relive life from a health perspective.

Do not ever be discouraged to create and manage your own well-being due to lack of time, tiredness, apathy or anything else which precludes you from taking daily action.

Personal Power means being awake and alive to the richness and fullness of life. It means approaching life with intensity, to create each moment with vigor and enthusiasm. For this is your natural birth right. However, far too many people believe otherwise - that the human form is designed to break down and not last beyond fifty years of age.

This is fallacy and perhaps an ideal that our western society has taught us over time. So starting afresh, from this moment onward, begin to view health and well-being with a new set of eyes. Create a new paradigm from which to live your life, using the *Personal Power* that will enable you to become more than what you want to be.

Ultimately, we create *Personal Power* by being present within our own bodies. The idea of being present is really about engaging our body's systems. Far too many people lead unhealthy lives, due largely to unhealthy rituals. When you live your life at the mercy of food or beverage addictions and cravings which own you, you are less present in your body and less engaged within the world.

Being free means liberating yourself from the need to resort to foods or beverages in order to feel better about yourself. As we will discuss in later chapters, many of these food cravings are rooted in an emotional disconnect.

Healthy individuals who *Navigate Life* have a sense of *Personal Power* insofar as they choose how and when to nourish their bodies. They are not subject to the same addictions as the majority of the world. Their emotional constitution is neither high nor low, but oscillates within the healthy range.

Navigating Life will allow you to become more acquainted with taking ownership of your body and your mind. I want you to create your sense of *Personal Power* and not have it thrust upon you by the high-tech marketing companies. When taking ownership of your *Personal Power*, you are empowered to make life choices and life decisions that are congruent with your **authentic nature.**Despite modern day marketing logic, *Health & Well-being* does not come in a bottle, a cream or potion. True wellness can only stem from within.

Your body has an innate wisdom, which regulates itself without the need of too much human interference. Note the biological rhythms and body systems which occur every second of every day in order to keep you alive, healthy and vibrant. Even the finest Swiss clocks need to be wound regularly in order to keep the parts moving. However, your human form does not require this type of mechanical maintenance. What it asks for and thrives on is being attuned to Mother Nature.

The final connecting principle on *The Power to Navigate Life* roadmap therefore becomes a Healthy and Vibrant Life. Returning to the example of the person who led an unhealthy lifestyle for much of their earlier years – ultimately the cells within the body are exhausted and breakdown, resulting in a host of health concerns. By the stage of life when a person is nearing midlife, reversing illness or disease becomes more difficult.

You will note that there is little vibrancy to their life. The individual at this stage gets caught up in the medical system and much of their retirement fund is paid toward doctors treating or managing illness. Once you get into the medical system, with declining health there is very little that you can do to get well again.

Our medical system has and will always be geared toward treating sickness, illness and disease. The medical model is based on diagnosing illness and treating it. Its main form of practice hinges on the presence of an illness for it to work. It is for this reason that the pharmaceutical industry collaborates with doctors to prescribe drugs, which in many cases are taken over the course of a person's life. It is my opinion that drug companies develop drugs to ease the symptoms, but not heal the malady. By doing so, they create a commodity.

The Power to Navigate Life is about empowering you with a sense of ownership of your own health. Your aim should be for you to never get caught up in the medical system so that you are better able to manage your health.

In my chiropractor's office there is a sign which adorns the fireplace, which I have studied for the last fifteen years as I visit her practice on a monthly basis. I recall in the earlier days that the message had very little significance for me. In time I have come to appreciate the message and what it means to the human race as we continue to evolve.

The quote is by Thomas Edison and reads:

> *The doctor of the future will give no medicine, but will interest her or his patients in the care of the human frame, in a proper diet and in the cause and prevention of disease.*

This quote is quite profound given it was framed over a century ago. My wish in the coming century is for health professionals to treat and cure illness and disease via nutrition alone.

We have already seen the emergence of holistic health modalities over the last fifty years. These have included the practices of naturopathy, homoeopathy, Chinese medicine and Reiki to name a few. Chinese medicine pre-dates Western medicine by thousands of years.

One downfall of Western medicine has been customizing people to the notion that healing is instantaneous. The proliferation of drug companies advising that we can heal any illness or disease via the use of drugs is possibly one of our greatest fallacies.

Author Dawson Church in his book Genie In Your Genes cites the following phrase: health is not an event, but a process which happens over time. Our greatest challenge in the modern era is going up against Western medicine that proclaims spontaneous healing via drugs. The irony of taking drugs to heal an illness or disease lies in the disconnect that one must continually take the drugs over a long period of time to see any benefit. Secondly, drugs must contain a side-effect, that affect bodily organs in order for them to heal a body system.

Holistic health practices on the other hand treat the body as an entire system. Rarely do holistic health practitioners prescribe potent drugs that affect an organ or a body system.

It is important to understand the difference between Eastern and Western health principles in order for you to make choices based on conscious awareness. Ultimately your long-term health and well-being rests in your ability to choose wisely.

Chapter Summary

- There are three main principles underlying *The Power to Navigate Life*: *Health & Well-being*, *Personal Power* and *Health & Vibrant Life*.

  » The first, Health and Well-being, is the springboard from which a prosperous life can emerge.

  » *Personal Power* enables us to create the ideal circumstances of our life. *Personal Power* means being awake and alive to the richness and fullness of life. It means approaching life with intensity, to create each moment with vigor and enthusiasm.

  » Healthy and Vibrant Life means living life full of passion and enthusiasm. It means being attuned to your emotional constitution and having the energy and vitality to make things happen.

- *The Power to Navigate Life* offers you an opportunity to experience an abundant, rich and prosperous life by developing sound health and well-being habits.

- Through awareness, you are able to choose how you treat your body. In doing so, your body will offer you a level of health and well-being that will enable you to experience a rich and fulfilling life.

CHAPTER TWO

Dimensions of The Power to Navigate Life

"So many people spend their health gaining wealth and then have to spend their wealth to regain their health."

A.J. Meteri

Four Channels

The Power to Navigate Life consists of four channels. The channels may be akin to a funnel. At the beginning of the funnel we have health and well-being. The next level is belief in a greater power. *Personal growth* is the next level down before reaching *self-awareness*.

Health and Wellbeing

In reviewing the last component of the dimensions of *The Power to Navigate Life*, the most compelling aspect of the program is attributed to the connection that *Health & Well-being* have to the other areas.

You have been given your body, your vessel from which to carry yourself through life. If the vessel or the container is sick or diseased then your journey is compromised. The biggest misconception that you have been told about health is that you can get it back. There is a famous quote by a Monk by the name of A.J. Meteri, which says,

"So many people spend their health gaining wealth and then have to spend their wealth to regain their health."

What is evident in the quote is that once we have used up our life force, it is virtually impossible to regain our level of health. You were born with a vital force of energy, this may be like being bestowed $1 million at the beginning of your life. Throughout the course of your life you spend that million dollars through various habits, rituals and practices. These may include a poor diet, high stress levels or lack of exercise. Once you have used up your health or your million dollars, it is very rare to recover or recoup that asset, since it has long gone. So the premise with Health and Well-being is to understand that you only have a finite amount of vital energy throughout your life. It is important that you choose the way in which you spend it.

Belief in a Greater Power

A belief in a greater power invites you to recognize that there is an energy source which is infinitely and creatively working on your behalf. This infinite source of energy is responsible for the beating of your heart, and the orchestration of millions of cells within your body. I like to look at this process as being similar to a school of fish swimming in perfect unison, when abruptly all turn and head off in a new direction. The synchronicity required to conduct such an action cannot be measured nor quantified through scientific data.

There is a source of energy available within the universe which is working on your behalf and serving you. When you begin to work with this greater intelligence and work with the universal laws that are available to you, you become the surfer surfing an endless wave. This belief in a greater source is not defined as a religion or cult, far too many people have been led to believe that they must be part of a religion in order to understand universal principles. This is the furthest thing from the truth, as your religion is contained within you right now.

You are the expression of life and that expression is making its way through you, every minute of the day. When you align yourself with this creative force, your life becomes a living miracle.

The second channel of dimensions of *The Power to Navigate Life* is an invitation to acknowledge that there is a greater force serving you and will continue to serve you for the rest of your life, as long as you learn to work with it.

Personal Growth

The purpose of *personal growth* within the channels of *Navigating Life* is to offer you a way to expand your mind and raise your consciousness. All disease and illness begins and manifests at the level of the mind. What you hold in your mind, in terms of thoughts and beliefs will be manifested at the physical level throughout your body.

Therefore, it is critical to raise your mental state by entertaining positive and affirming thoughts on a continual basis. When we contemplate thoughts about any aspect of our body, which moves away from nature, the results is pain, disease or illness. In his book, *The Mind-Body Prescription*, Dr. John Sarno attributes the effects of anxiety and anger to a condition known as TMS, or Tension Myositis Syndrome. He postulates that our thoughts drive our emotional state, which consequently affects our physiology.

Personal growth invites you to be acutely aware of your predominant thoughts. When you are aware of your thoughts, you become the observer of the thoughts, rather than being engaged with the thought and owning the thought. There are many eastern practices that state that you are not the product of your thoughts, nor are you the thought itself. Rather you are the observer of the thought. When you appreciate this knowledge, every thought that you entertain about your body, whether it be of sickness, illness or otherwise, can be viewed from a larger perspective. You can view these thoughts as an observer, rather than becoming invested in the thought.

Self-Awareness

Socrates said, "know thyself." In knowing oneself, you are able to make more informed and conscious decisions about your life and about your health. People who possess *Self-Awareness* have an ability to choose consciously, rather than existing in constant state of response to cause and effect situations.

By acquiring *Self-Awareness*, you make conscious decisions and choices that are in alignment with your deepest self. This authentic self already knows what to do for it has an infinite intelligence which was bequeathed at the time of your birth. I like to think of this analogy as that of a tree. A tree does not have to be told when to shed its leaves in season, for it does so with perfect timing and precision as the seasons change. A tree knows when to cast shade to protect the grass beneath it or to shield animals from the sun during the warmer months. A tree never looks to the sun or Mother Nature for advice. It knows what to do day in, day out.

So when you become self-aware, there is a tendency to go inward and become aware of not only physical sensations, but mental and emotional states as well. Far too many people live their lives unaware of subtle shifts or changes within their bodies. It is not until a disease or illness takes hold that they notice this shift occur.

Therefore, the aim of *Self-awareness* is a dimension of *Navigating Life* to help you have a greater awareness of yourself. The more aware you become, the better you are able to make conscious and informed decisions in any area of your life.

In the coming chapters I will introduce you to concepts and principles that are the foundation to becoming more self-aware. Like any practice in life, you must put these principles into practice in your daily life.

Self-awareness is serving you at every moment of your life. When you choose to dial into its frequency, you will notice subtle changes beginning to emerge.

Chapter Summary

- *The Power to Navigate Life* consists of four channels. The channels may be likened to a funnel.

- At the beginning of the funnel we have health and well-being. The next level is belief in a greater power. *Personal growth* is the next level down before reaching *self-awareness.*

- A belief in a greater power is the understanding that there is an energy source which is infinitely and creatively working on your behalf. This infinite source of energy is responsible for the beating of your heart, and the orchestration of millions of cells within your body.

- The purpose of *personal growth* within the channels of *Navigating Life* is to offer you a way to expand your mind and raise your consciousness.

- All disease and illness begins and manifests at the level of the mind. *Personal Growth* invites you to be aware of the nature of your thoughts.

- *Self-Awareness* allows you to choose consciously, rather than existing in constant state of response to cause and effect situations.

- Through *Self-Awareness*, you make conscious decisions and choices that are in alignment with your deepest self.

- The aim of *Self-awareness* as a dimension of *Navigating Life* is to help you have a greater awareness of yourself. The more aware you become, the better you are able to make conscious and informed decisions in any area of your life.

Life's Roadmap

Parked versus Navigate Life

"Health is not an event, but a process which happens over time."
Dawson Church

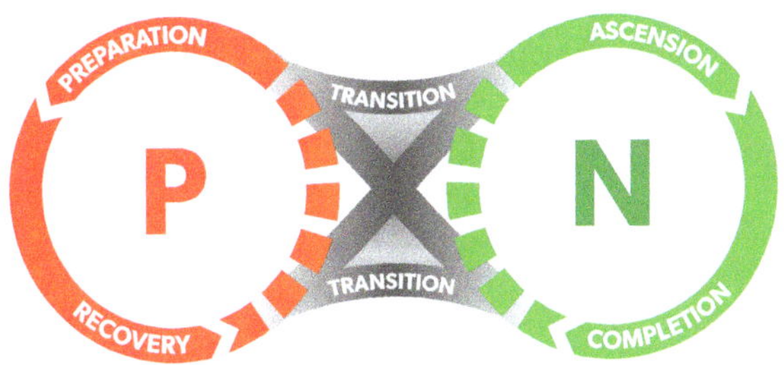

Working with the concept of *Navigating* versus *Parked* as a symbol of the expression of life, I began to see two components to it. The graphic shown above represents two components of life. The inspiration for this symbol was taken from the yin and yang symbol.

It is a map of life, which is cyclical in nature. You will note that there is a flowing of energy from one side of the chart to the other. There is no stagnation at any point. On the left hand side, represented in red is the *Parked* station. The top of the *Parked* circle is represented by Preparation. If you follow the arrow in a counter clockwise direction you arrive at

Recovery at the bottom.

Following on from recovery, there is a dotted section which makes up a complete circle. Immediately after recovery there is a grey area in between, known as transition. This transition area is indicative of the transitions that we undergo in life. What is compelling about this chart is that it allows us to view our life from a bigger picture, rather than becoming invested in the small details and aspects of our life. When we view life from this perspective, we can see that there are no mistakes in life, but rather movement of energy from one area to the other.

I represented *Parked* purposely in red to highlight its metaphysical relationship to being stuck or parked in a car. When you think of being *parked*, there is a stagnant energy about it as you are not going anywhere. You are enclosed in inner space and unable to move freely. This is the feeling that comes to us at moments of our life when we feel there is no direction or purpose to our life. This is not necessarily a bad thing. What I would like to represent in this diagram is one of two components:

Being *Parked* represents the transition to the next phase, which is *Navigating Life*. We repeat the cycle of being *Parked* and stay within the red circle until we have learnt the lesson.

It is worth noting and understanding that the process of life is cyclical and if we are to create our own *Personal Power* and lead a rich and rewarding life, it is essential that we know where we are within this cycle.

The *Preparation* phase on the left hand side represents a learning point for us. It illustrates something that we are ready to learn, or understand before we transition to the next phase. A good way to understand preparation is that sometimes we may have experienced a number of setbacks or failures in our attempt to pursue or attain a goal. When entrenched in the day to day running of our life, it may appear as a setback, when in fact it is a preparation for the next phase that will soon follow.

The next phase that follows can be seen at the bottom of the red circle on the left-hand side. This is known as *Recovery*. The *Recovery* phase is almost the free intermediary stage before we transition to the green *Navigating* side. When we are in the *Recovery* phase, the opportunity to learn our lessons becomes invaluable before we proceed to our next life's lesson. Many people feel like skipping this stage in order to attain whatever goal they have been working toward. For example, if your goal was to find a new job with a rewarding career prospect, you may have stumbled on what appeared to be roadblocks and unsuccessful job interviews. These *Recovery* phases provide sound learning before you transition into the *Ascension* phase of the *Navigating* cycle as illustrated in green on the right-hand side of the diagram.

The grey area in between represents the transitory phase that one experiences during the course of their life. This is not seen as good or bad and it must be highlighted that the diagram is not indicative of good or bad circumstances, rather events that dictate the course of life.

Recall a moment of your life when you were in transition. This may have included leaving a relationship that ran its course. The relationship may have been personal or business. You may have seen the end of a job and decided on another career. During this time, you decided to take some time to investigate other options for further study or self-improvement. You may have been unsure as to where your future was heading at the time. This constitutes the *Transition* phase, since there is an element of the unknown – this may be viewed as a positive phase, for the excitement and unfolding of events in the future will dictate the course of your life.

The point worth noting is that you do not become invested in any one area of life. Everything is continually in transition. Life is perpetual and cyclical in motion. The diagram serves as a reminder or compass to chart your journey. When you view life from this perspective, you will come to appreciate that there are no mistakes and that everything that happens to you, flows through you. You become the conduit and expression of life, for there are no mistakes in the journey, which ultimately allows you to arrive at your desired destination.

Transitional phases within life are essential components insofar as they allow us to prepare for the next phase in life. If we look to Mother Nature, we notice that transitions are also evident. Spring precedes summer as does autumn to winter. The seasonal changes allow for different cycles in nature. There is harmony in unity and there is perpetual motion that is forever taking place if we allow the process to unfold by removing ourselves from the drama.

Moving onto the right side of the diagram, we are now *Navigating Life*. When *Navigating Life* you are in command of the life process and there is harmony and unity in every action. Hopefully, all the preceding events that took place in the *Parked* and *Transition* states have now been secured, allowing you to enjoy the fruits of your labor.

You will note that the top of the circle in the *Navigating* aspect is denoted by the word *Ascension*. The *Ascension* phase is that aspect of life when you acquire or gained a new learning or an understanding. It might be that something had to close in the *Parked* state in order for something new to open and reveal itself. Sometimes these things might include relationships, whether they are personal, romantic or business or even career or financial.

The key understanding here is that by relinquishing an issue or something falling away, allows you to open the door to something new. For most people however, when they are entrenched in the drama of their life, they often see a negative event as such. The truth of the matter is that life is far more whole and complete when we allow ourselves to step back from the entire picture and allow the process to reveal itself. In doing so we see the gift that had to take place, and that it is an essential part of allowing us to arrive at our destination.

Hopefully, by viewing life from this perspective you begin to see that all your thoughts, deeds and actions are evolving for your highest good. .

Once we transition through the *Ascension* phase, we move on to the *Completion* phase. There is no set time between these phases. For some it might take weeks, for others it might be months or even years. The key element here is not to be tied or bound by time, for the Universe works in mysterious ways and in a timeline not of our own accord. It is at this point we learn to relinquish and handover, with no need to control life or events, by becoming less invested in the outcome and more attuned to the lessons that we learn. As the lessons we learn ultimately create the person that we become.

It is clear that there are steps in life that are essential to your personal growth. Fast tracking these experiences leads to lessons which are missed. These lessons form vital tools and resources to help you Navigate Life effectively.

Chapter Summary

- The concept of *Navigating* versus *Parked* as a symbol illustrates the expression of life, of which there are two components to it.

- It is a map of life, which is cyclical in nature. There is a flowing of energy from one side of the chart to the other. The energy is constant and moves from one form to another depending on your current state of reality.

- *Parked* is shown in red to highlight its metaphysical relationship to being stuck or parked in a car. Think about the relationship of being 'stuck in traffic' or 'stuck at the lights.'

- The *Transition* phase in between, is an element of the unknown – this may be viewed as a positive phase, for the excitement and unfolding of events in the future will dictate the course of your life. Do not view this transitory phase as unwanted.

- *Navigating Life* means you are in command of the life process and there is harmony and unity in every action.

- The *Navigating Life* diagram serves as a compass to chart your journey throughout life.

- When you view life from this perspective, you will come to appreciate that there are no mistakes and that everything that happens to you, flows through you.

- The chart is therefore a representation of your current state of reality and a means by which to chart your future destiny.

CHAPTER FOUR

A Comparative View

A *Window of Opportunity*

"Change the way you look at things and the things you look at change."

Dr Wayne Dyer

PARKED	NAVIGATING
You view circumstances as a challenge instead of an opportunity to learn and grow.	You act through inspiration, not perspiration.
You are frustrated in relationships, perhaps looking for a way out. The other person is the problem – not you.	You appreciate the world reflects back your current reality. Change within and without follows.
You may have a cynical outlook about the world, since there is always evidence to substantiate it.	You are optimistic as a result of your beliefs; you attract the ideal circumstances in life.
Money is hard to come by. You live from pay check to pay check. It seems to slip through your fingers.	You are a conscious creator. Money flows into your life easily and effortlessly when you are in alignment with your purpose.
You are scared and removed from anything which you cannot see. "See it before you believe it."	You are open and receptive to the flow of information, ideas & events in your life. "You believe it, and then begin to see evidence of it materialize."

In the diagram above we see there are two columns depicting the qualities of life when viewed from the *Parked* or *Navigating* perspectives. If you read over the *Parked* section, you will be aware that viewing the world from this perspective equates to an experience that is stagnant, blunt, and static. I have purposely labeled the columns in red and green to identify the red with being **static** and the green depicting the **dynamic energy** of life.

Each moment life creates itself anew. When we are open and receptive to what life brings, instead of resisting and fighting, we begin to cooperate with life. But life will always win when we attempt to oppose it. Our opposition to life stems from our need to suit the outside world to our needs. Something inside of us says that if things were different on the outside, then we would be happy and content on the inside. It rarely ever works out that way, for we are attempting to base our internal happiness on external conditions, which are often beyond our control.

Another way to look at it is from the perspective that although we cannot change external conditions, **you can control your inner world and how you respond to it**. Let us look at this statement from the view of an athlete.

A skilled and trained runner needs to adjust himself to suit a variety of race conditions. He cannot possibly compete at international level and in different countries with only limited race prowess. A successful athlete learns to race and train in a variety of conditions, locally and internationally. In doing so, he becomes well accustomed to a variety of conditions that help him to become a stronger and prized competitor.

Our lives are not dissimilar to that of athletes. We are faced with challenges every day. These challenges are not coincidental or unfortunate. They come to us in order to allow us to grow and evolve into a superior person who is capable of withstanding anything life throws our way. Life, whilst rewarding as it is, is nonetheless challenging at the best of times. Returning to the analogy of the athlete, it becomes essential that we grow and evolve so that we are well equipped to face and deal with life's hurdles.

Now, let us examine the table starting from the left hand side when one is in the *Parked* state. Notice in the first box, when we are in the *Parked* state we view circumstances as a challenge instead of an opportunity to learn and grow. One of the greatest gifts I have acquired in this experience is the ability to see that everything that transpires in my life does so for the unfolding of my greatest good. Most people's challenges lie in their inability to see what is before them is actually a gift—a gift wrapped up as a challenge.

We could not possibly grow as individuals if life were easy all of the time. Recalling the athlete, the more challenges the athlete is faced with, the stronger and faster he becomes. If we navigate by similar thinking, we grow into circumstances rather than trying to force them to happen.

Understand this:
> The life challenges you currently face, whether they be financial, relationship, career or other, are calling you to face your challenges with a new mind and a new outlook. When you raise your level of consciousness, your level of thinking raises to view problems as opportunities.

In contrast, if you look to the box on the right-hand side under *Navigating* you will note that the person who *Navigates Life* acts from inspiration rather than perspiration. Inspired people have more energy to make things happen.
> The word **inspired** is intentionally used in contrast to the term motivated, as the term **motivated** implies stimulus from an external source, as opposed to being **inspired** from within.

I like to look at inspiration from this perspective. Consider the great Renaissance painter Michelangelo. I do not think Michelangelo ever had to be motivated to get up each morning to paint the Sistine Chapel. Michelangelo was inspired to create these pieces of art. People who are inspired have an inner purpose, an inner calling. I personally believe this inner call is the expression of life—the Universe seeking to express itself. People who are inspired rarely get tired and are enthusiastic about their mission or purpose. They cannot wait to get up each morning and be of service.

Let us look at the second box within the *Parked* table on the left-hand side to examine another life view. In a *Parked* state, you may view a relationship as frustrating, believing the other person is always the issue not you. The point is that *Parked* people attempt to change their external world to suit their internal world. Unfortunately, life is too complex to wish that our external world will succumb to our wants, needs or desires.

In order to look at this from a higher perspective, you need to change your *internal* reference of your *external* world. In this example, it is worth noting that when we are in an intimate relationship, our partner is effectively mirroring back aspects of our personality, which we either repress or dislike. The fact that it pushes our buttons is evidence enough that we identify with an unfavorable quality within ourselves. The key is not so much to fix the problem, as to become aware that you possess this quality. Through awareness and conscious will, you are able to heal that part of your nature and create a more fulfilling and joyful intimate relationship.

The answer to any of our troubles is revealed by turning inward and reflecting upon the nature of that disturbance. Interactions with our partners sometimes evoke mental or emotional sensitivities associated with childhood trauma or past experiences we have repressed. However, denying an aspect of ourselves could result from an unconscious process. If we were harmed emotionally when we were young, our minds unconsciously repress the pain, possibly as a protective measure. It is only later in adult life, when our mind has developed, that many of our childhood beliefs and programs return.

Those *Navigating life*, acknowledge that the world is reflecting back their current state of reality. Change within and without follows.

Change the way you look at things and the things you look at change, is a well-known spiritual saying which proclaims our capacity to be conscious creators of our life circumstances. Those *Navigating* understand that the world outside is a reflection of their inner world. Instead of trying to fix things on the outside they tend to their inner world and heal mental or emotional states which are not in alignment with their desires.

People who are *Navigating* are continually realigning themselves to obtain the highest level of joy and fulfillment. Pilots do the same thing when flying; as the plane flies toward its destination, its satellite navigation system is repeatedly updating in order keep the plane on course to reach the desired destination. Likewise, those *Navigating* look toward their inner world in order to adjust and create their outer world experiences.

The *Parked* vs. *Navigating* comparative diagram illustrates the respective life views of each state. The key is to never stay stuck in one area and to recognize when we are stagnant and not moving forward. When *Navigating*, we have the ability to self-correct: to steer ourselves into the future, to curtail regret.

Chapter Summary

- The table illustrates the qualities of life from the *Parked* or *Navigating* perspectives.

- The *Parked* vs. *Navigating* comparative diagram illustrates the respective life views of each state.

- The key to *Navigating Life* is to never stay stuck in one area and to recognize when you are stagnant and not moving forward. The table comparison serves as a gauge, providing you immediate feedback on your present life.

- When we are open and receptive to what life brings, instead of resisting and fighting, we begin to cooperate with life.

- Although we cannot change external conditions, you can control your inner world and how you respond to it.

- We are faced with challenges every day which are not coincidental or unfortunate. They help us to grow and evolve into one who is capable of withstanding anything life throws our way.

- Your current life challenges, whether they be financial, relationship, career or other, are inviting you to view them with a new mind and a new outlook.

- When you raise your level of consciousness, your level of thinking raises to view problems as opportunities.

- People who are inspired have an inner purpose, an inner calling.

- This inner call is the expression of life – the Universe seeking to express itself through you.

- *Parked* people attempt to change their external world to suit their internal world.

- People who *Navigate Life* act from inspiration rather than perspiration.

- Inspired people have more energy to make things happen rather than bemoan their current state of reality.

- The answer to any of our troubles is naturally to retreat within and reflect upon where the disturbance is coming from.

- Our relationship with our partners sometimes bring out mental or emotional issues connected with our childhood trauma or past experiences we have repressed.

- Those Navigating life understand that the world outside is a reflection of their inner world.

- Instead of trying to fix things on the outside, tend to your inner world and heal any mental or emotional states which are not in alignment with your desires.

CHAPTER FIVE
A Health Perspective

Navigate Your Health

"Just because you're not sick doesn't mean you're healthy"

Author Unknown

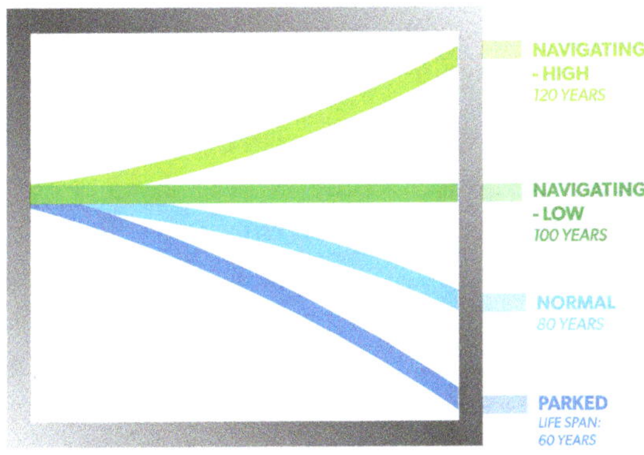

Many present day problems stem from poor health. Our thoughts, emotions, and interactions with the outside world are reflected in the health and well-being of our bodies. Our cells thrive on being in the highest state of health in order to bring us the fullest life experiences. Unfortunately, we were not born with instruction manuals for the bodies.

Through trial and error we learn to tend and care for our bodies, though sadly, many of us choose to put toxic thoughts, emotions and substances inside. Over time, the toxic overload incapacitates the normal function of our bodies, thereby disrupting the natural state of health.

I have seen far too many times, people whom have intentionally abused their bodies through repeated toxic behavior and stressful states. Although having treated their bodies so poorly, they still expected peak performance. Not even a well-intentioned machine has the capacity to perform at the highest level without the correct maintenance and quality lubricants.

Fortunately, your body is not a machine and does not require petroleum lubrication and upgrades. What it does require is the higher source nutrients and continued caring maintenance. A body that receives this will continue to thrive and maintain a high state of homoeostasis, meaning balanced health. Given that we are living in a modern world, the stresses that are imposed upon us repeatedly drain our health, well-being and vitality. The ageing process is accelerated every single day from the moment we wake up until our head hits the pillow each evening.

It is vital that in order to *Navigate Life*, we need to take ownership of our health as the highest priority. In doing so, we de-accelerate the ageing process while our body remains healthy, vital and well. Given modern convention, most people are inclined to believe that taking care of their body is a chore and for this reason skip a great deal of the process involved on a day-to-day basis. Your body is a vital organism which needs to be attended to and cared for in order that it carry you through life, enabling you to experience a richness toward life.

Many people hold an inaccurate belief that the body breaking down is part of the ageing process. In the Western world we believe that as we reach our forties and fifties, that ageing is inevitable and our body begins to break down. It is during this period that many people begin to experience a host of illnesses and even general malaise. Digestive issues with chronic joint pain and inflammation are the leading cause of early warning signs that the body is experiencing a breakdown in its natural rhythm.

It is around this time that people seek the advice of their medical practitioner, who with all good intentions prescribe drugs to treat the ailing organ or body system. The predicament with Western medicine however, is that in order for a drug to have an effect on a body system, it must also have a counter effect; one symptom is alleviated, whilst another surfaces.

Do not get me wrong, I am not denouncing Western medicine. In fact, it is Western medicine itself that has contributed toward people living longer, thanks in large to advances in surgery. However, one cannot rely on Western medicine alone to maintain health and well-being. It is essential that you take ownership of your health through conscious effort.

History has shown us that lifestyle plays a tremendous role in longevity and quality of life. My personal interest in health and well-being resulted from my own illness. As I began to understand the steps to achieving radiant health and well-being, I became deeply intrigued with longevity. It was around this time that I began studying the populations of the world, that live well beyond their nineties and into their hundreds.

I soon discovered documented populations living well into their nineties and beyond in present day. A list of such groups follows:

- Vilcabamba, Ecuador

- Hunza region, Pakistan

- Southern Russia

- Okinawa, Japan

Among these communities, those members living beyond their nineties are well respected and revered within their communities. For some reason, in Western society, as a person ages there is a tendency toward seeing them as less able. Western society is influenced heavily by media and the relative disposability of everything and inundating our culture with imagines of youth.

Ageing, therefore, must be viewed in a new context in our society if we are to approach the latter years of our life with a similar degree of joy, health and abundance. I do, however, feel that there is a shift occurring, and as we enter the next decade, we stand on the precipice of the union of spirit and matter. As our consciousness continues to evolve and expand, we will begin to harness our inner potential and wisdom, and our focus will begin to move away from facade.

The health perspective diagram shown on previously illustrates four areas of relative health, based upon a *Parked* or *Navigating* framework. Starting at the bottom in the dark blue we see that a person who thinks with a *Parked* mindset is likely to only live to sixty years of age. If we make assumptions here, given the information that we have addressed earlier, we can assume that a person who is *Parked* generally has a tendency toward negative thinking. These thoughts are not particularly orientated toward a positive mind set and for this reason the body will represent what is held at the level of the mind.

A person with a *Parked* mind set will generally entertain the same repeated thoughts and will not be conscious of their own thought pattern. It is only once the level of consciousness is raised that we begin to impact our bodies in positive ways.

While this shift in thought tends to have an effect on other areas of our lives, behaviors that the *Parked* person exhibits may not be conducive to a healthy lifestyle. This may include the use of excessive alcohol, lack of exercise, poor nutrition and lifestyle choices. Whilst this is not always the case, the purpose of this exercise is to create a framework from which to move someone out of a *Parked* state and into a *Navigating* state.

It is worth mentioning here that while you may be *Navigating* in one area of your life, such as career, you may be stagnant and remain *Parked* in another area of your life such as relationships. And I stress here that there is no right or wrong and that the person evaluating themselves should not look unfavorably upon your current life circumstances. Rather, this book is designed to help you evaluate and gain a greater awareness of those areas of your life that require your attention. In doing so, you are able to act swiftly to bring about changes before it is too late. Many of these changes, especially relating to health and well-being, should be made sooner rather than later. For when disease begins to manifest, the body will give clear warning signs that something is out of balance. The purpose of understanding whether you are in a *Parked* or *Navigating* state is to take immediate action, steering toward better health.

As we move up to the next level which is marked as *Normal*, with a corresponding life span of eighty years we find the age-range where most people in Western society aspire to live. It is commonly believed that living to eighty years of age is a long life and whilst I am not discounting this, I feel that many of the ailments experienced in "old age" are acquired in middle age. To enjoy life more fully, we have to be conscious of the bodies capacity to age healthily and treat the body accordingly in earlier stages of life.

During my investigation of ageing, I discovered that those people who live beyond 100 years all had a common set of practices and habits that contributed towards their longevity. Many of these included the minimal consumption of meat, regular walking and exercise, social gatherings, a healthy and positive outlook towards life and a refusal to let life slow them down.

The other common theme that was noticed among centenarians and beyond, was the rich lives they led working on the land. Whilst the thought of living a physically productive life at 100 may seem quaint, the active lifestyles of the centenarians was paired with long periods of inactivity during the winter months. This was attributed to a lack of electricity in their region, which meant sleeping for most of the day and staying indoors. Largely, this is a testament to the value of rest and balance. In retrospect I believe that in the Western world we have a pretty good balance given the hectic lives we lead. Read more of this philosophy from John Robbin's book, *Healthy at 100*. It would be good for you to understand the key areas from centenarians and put these habits and practices in your own life.

In recent times, researchers have come to a greater understanding that what a person holds in mind in relation to a belief system, regarding ageing, is a strong indicator on how long that person will live. Your belief system exists within every cell of your body. I have spoken about how our thoughts influence chemical reactions within our bodies. What we think about, we bring about. It is no secret that as we begin to harness the power of the mind, it has a ripple effect on our human physiology.

Candace Pert wrote her book, *Molecules of Emotion*, about the body being the subconscious mind. Dr. Pert conducted numerous studies over the years with in-depth research to draw conclusions that your body has a mind of its own. This is evident, from the digestive system, otherwise known as the enteric nervous system. The enteric nervous system has a mind of its own. You have probably heard the adage "a gut feeling", which pertains to having an intuitive feeling in response to external stimuli. Many artists, musicians and creative people often talk about this "gut feeling" or "going with one's gut."

What they are talking about in this case is the ability to feel a situation rather than mentally process it.

Research has indicated that the gut maintains an autonomous relationship to the brain. Scientists have indicated that if one were to cut the main nerve supplying the digestive system (the Vagus nerve) that the digestive system would still function of its own accord. They reached this conclusion after conducting experiments where they believed the neurotransmitter serotonin was thought to be manufactured in the brain. Conclusive research has shown that 80% of serotonin is manufactured in the mucosa lining of the digestive system.

Evidently, approximately 80% of your immune system is also contained within the gut. It is for this reason that what you eat and how you nourish your body relates to the health and well-being of your immune system. If you have ever eaten food which did not agree with you, whether through contamination or an allergic reaction, you will have noted the speed at which your body worked to expel the offending food. Your body continually works to maintain perfect unison and harmony together with your other body systems.

Our bodies are composed of entire networks of organic substances. All body systems are inexorably linked and therefore cannot be isolated nor treated in isolation. When you begin to view your body as a whole organic system, rather than attending to individual parts, health and well-being become expressions of that thinking. Eastern medicine, which predates Western medicine, views the body as an entire system.

The body system fully functioning can live until eighty years of age, which is what most people have come to expect. To assist the body in its longevity, we must avoid certain toxic behaviors and habits that include excessive drinking, alcohol and drug abuse while maintaining a well-balanced and healthy lifestyle. I have seen others achieve this by merely attending to their nutrition alone, without including exercise in their life, which is somewhat adverse to what the heavy exercise culture endorsed in the West, as many surrogate exercise for "healthy lifestyle" in lieu of addressing nutritional needs. When exercise becomes chronic, such as excessive cardio, the body begins running on adrenaline and in doing so inhibits and shuts down organ function in order to preserve life. Exercise should be used to complement a sound nutritional program, to balance life.

Health problems in the Western world can also be attributed to an emotional disconnect of our external reality from the internal world. A large proportion of people seem to have fluctuating emotions which are linked to outside events. When our emotions are linked to learned childhood behaviors, it becomes increasingly challenging for us to navigate a healthy way of being.

For example, many childhood programs relate to reward systems centered on food. You may have grown up in a household where deserts, cake and chocolate were frequently eaten after a meal or used as a form of celebratory event to mark an achievement or reward. In doing so one associates an emotional connection to a reward and an event due to the emotions that it provides a person and evidently takes this behavior into their adult life.

It is for this reason that when things do not go as planned in adult life, people often resort to various forms of foods in order to seek pleasure. Whilst I do not see any long-term danger in doing so, the potential for this to become a recurring habit leading to excessive weight gain or other health conditions is a cause for concern.

Navigating Life in relation to your health and well-being, means that you are in conscious control of *how* and *what* with your body is nourished. People who are conscious and aware tend to choose foods that are in alignment with their highest potential. They tend not to have strong habits and cravings toward any particular type of food because they are aware of their emotional constitutions. They do not use food as a means of seeking comfort when times are tough. Instead, through conscious awareness they seek meaning and understanding on how they can attend to any emotional disturbance in the body.

Knowing oneself becomes an essential component toward living a joyous, prosperous and healthy life. People who act unconsciously are not aware of the thought processes and therefore are unable to take action to remedy a situation which may be out of control. This may relate to nutrition, exercise, sleep or any other facet of one's health and well-being. The key is to recognize when a pattern of behavior continues to show up in our lives and then subsequently take immediate conscious action in order to find out the root cause of that behavior.

I do not subscribe to the notion that you must deprive yourself of anything, in order to gain a satisfying result. It is important to ask yourself a series of questions to find out *what* you desire and examine *why* you desire that thing/experience. When you have a clear understanding of your wants, needs and desires it becomes far more pleasant and simpler to create a roadmap toward fulfillment.

Experiencing setbacks while creating your optimal health and well-being is inevitable and part of the process. DO NOT BE DISCOURAGED. The important lesson to gain from the experience is the understanding of how to circumvent and work around these setbacks in the future. Fumbling along the journey is part of the learning experience. Without setbacks, we would undoubtedly repeat many of our destructive and toxic habits which were created long ago.

The next level in the health perspective is *Navigating Low (100 years)*, which is indicated on the diagram as 100 years of age. In order for one to reach this level, it is important to approach your health and well-being program from a higher perspective. This might include abstaining from certain foods such as grains, dairy products and anything containing sugar. It might be that you switch from physical exercise to more meditative types of movement, such as yoga, Tai Chi or simply walking. Meditation is normally added if a person has not meditated previously, since this practice can benefit both mind and body.

Of the many books that have been written about people living to 100 and beyond, they all seem to indicate a preference toward a gentler way of life, both outwardly and inwardly. My personal belief is that when we learn to live in tune with nature, we harness our genetic potential to activate our true genetic expression. The further we move away from nature in how we nourish our body and also through chronic exercise and stress, the less health and vitality we have in our later years.

In contrast, gentler exercises, which are low impact and focus on improving muscle tone and bone strength and also posture and flexibility, may be viewed as more effective exercises that can be performed in later years. I recall working with a client some years ago who at the time was aged sixty-five. This client had grown up with four other brothers who were all active from a young age, having participated in sport regularly. The client showed interest toward the arts and never really undertook any health or exercise regime and in fact shunned going to health clubs. It was not until his mid-forties that he began to take exercise seriously and so began a passion of learning to manage his health and well-being by performing exercises that promoted long-term health and well-being.

You are never too old to start a health program. The key is always to start small and gain momentum by participating in activities that are fun and enjoyable. A good way to start an exercise program is to take advantage of the social settings that are available today. It is been shown that when people gather together in social circumstances for a common cause, i.e.

weight loss to improve health and well-being, the likelihood of sticking to the program and achieving results increases tenfold. We are social beings and for that reason we participate in programs that are fun, enjoyable and socially rewarding.

I think it is important to decide at an early stage of life whether we to want to live a long and healthy life. I do not believe you need to buy into the notion that as you age your health will deteriorate. We are now living longer than ever before thanks to the advances in medicine. Albeit, whilst medicine allows us to live longer; it can be to the detriment of having to take medication during the latter part of one's life.

It is important that you understand that you have the genetic equivalent and capacity to live a long and healthy life. Probably the only reason that you believe that your health declines is attributed to media and marketing campaigns, which have told us that we are of little use as we age. Indigenous tribes and cultures that still thrive today do not have this concept of an ageing being equated to a decline in vitality. It is only our Western phenomena that have been impregnated into our minds.

It is worth mentioning that statistics indicate that those who retire normally have a decline in health within a decade of their retirement. Ironically, the centenarians were found to still be working performing labor well into their nineties and beyond. Many of them attribute their daily walks and regular activity to their longevity (adapted from John Robbins book, *Healthy at 100*). I think we need to question what we have been told in terms of being the ideal lifestyle and re-examine it, if we wish to live a long, healthy and prosperous life.

Perhaps, if people engaged in careers that were rewarding and stimulating, they would not retire so young. The concept of retirement goes well beyond a physical level. There is a sense that one is retiring from life, almost as though they are checking out. What if you pursued a passion from a young age that allowed you to continue doing that job or career well into your seventies and eighties? There are many people living today of that age who still continue to enjoy their career and serve others in the process. Remember earlier that I mention Candace Pert whose work into the molecules of emotion reveals that the body was the subconscious mind. Your body knows and interprets every thought and emotion that takes place in your mind and body. There is no lying or no way that you can deceive your body with illegitimate thoughts.

I recall a conversation with a notable physician many years ago. I asked him his advice about disease and illness since he had specialized in the area of diabetes. One remarkable thing that I remember was in relation to how we treat our bodies in the early stages of our adult life. His contention, based on years of experience was how one chooses to nutritionalize, and look after their health and well-being in their twenties and thirties, normally marks the way in which that person will live out their fifties and beyond.

He continued by saying people who abused their bodies in the early stages of their adult life, which might have included a poor diet, smoking, lack of exercise and excessive drinking normally paid the price via illness and disease in the later stage of their life.

He went on to conclude that in many instances, disease and illness takes anywhere between a decade or two to manifest itself throughout the body. For some reason we believe that if this person has a poor diet, and there are no external symptoms of illness or disease, then they must be healthy.

The opposite of this is true. For a healthy body, any toxins or unhealthy food that is consumed will be quickly and effectively disposed of via one of the four detoxification organs of the body. A healthy, thriving cell will remove toxins immediately once they enter the cell. They do not get trapped within the cell and deprive the body of immunity, which therefore causes a host of health related symptoms. A healthy cell is designed to thrive at the highest level and detoxify the body.

A good analogy of the cell working in perfect harmony is shown in the following context. Your body is like a helium balloon, it is continually striving to maintain the highest state of homoeostasis and equilibrium. Unfortunately, due to the many toxins and the nature of our modern life, your body cells become overburdened and taxed in such a way that the cell is inhibited in the way that it performs its job.

As the saying goes: *junk in, junk out.* The quality of the nutrients that are consumed by the human body are of the utmost importance, since the body is designed to draw nutrients, vitamins and minerals from the foods you ingest which form the building blocks of many functions.

Obesity is not an intended function of Mother Nature's design. You need only look to the animal kingdom to see how effectively and effortlessly Mother Nature operates. It is rare to see animals living in the wild that are obese or overweight. For these animals are in their natural environment, operating within the system of evolution that nature intended. Obesity in that case is a man-made problem, largely caused by our inability to work with Mother Nature.

When you align yourself with the essential laws of healthy nutrition, your body will thrive and continually do so at the highest state of health and well-being with minimal effort. Nature does not complicate what it can simplify and if we look to the plant and animal world, this is no more evidence in the simplicity at which nature effortlessly operates.

If it is your intention to live a long, prosperous and healthy life then you must educate yourself with the knowledge and resources required to make that journey possible. At various stages of your life you will undergo many changes that will herald the way in which your body thrives. For many, this may include the dietary changes, exercise habits and undertaking a form of holistic health practice that may include: meditation, yoga, or perhaps some other form of lower intensity movement, which is less physically demanding on the human body.

These evolutionary changes will occur at certain times of your life when you are ready to adopt better ways of living. Be open and receptive to listening to your body and being in tune to what your body is asking of you. Being receptive to these changes means having awareness toward nurturing your human form in another way. If you have always run long distances as a form of exercise and your knee joints are beginning to wear out, then it may be time to re-examine a different form of exercise that is less demanding on your joints, yet still offers you the same feelings that come from running.

Many people get stuck into habitual patterns of behavior that they have pursued during the course of their life. Often, these behaviors may not be the best suited to toward maintaining long-term health and well-being. I believe it is essential to re-examine if our habits are drawing us closer toward lasting health or depriving us of that goal.

There is no great satisfaction living beyond eighty years of age when having to rely on medication for the day-to-day function of many physiological processes within the human body.

As we move on to the next level, within the health perspective diagram, we reach the 120 milestone. There are various suggestions that have been made by a number of older people who claim to be 130 years of age. Scientists examining these people discovered that it was unlikely that they lived to this age and that there was no possible way of proving their longevity, given the fact that there is no documentation of these people's births.

The oldest known person is believed to have lived 122 years and there is documented evidence to substantiate their age. This gives hope and sheds light on the possibility that those human beings have the capacity to live well beyond their 100 years of age, given the right environment and the right condition. I believe that we are on the precipice of a new era as we come to a new understanding in Western medicine that enables us to live a longer life span. As mentioned earlier, living longer may entail a new set of problems that doctors and scientists may have to tackle at some stage.

Research scientists believe that living beyond 100 years of age signifies having a particular genetic disposition insofar as there are not many people with the right genetic constitution that are able to live well beyond their 100 years. My belief is that the environment needs to be conducive to sustaining a way of life that allows an individual to thrive on a day-to-day basis. Many of the people who live beyond 100 do so in an environment that is normally at altitude and free of the pollution that makes up modern-day living in cities.

We need to strike a balance to create the ideal circumstances for humans to thrive physically, mentally and emotionally as we create new technologies that paved the way for increased lifespan.

The diagram clearly illustrates 120 years as *Navigating High*. This may be viewed as an aspirational milestone or one in which we may learn to work toward as we begin to expand what is physically possible in human evolution.

Chapter Summary

- Our cells thrive on being in the highest state of health in order to bring us the fullest life experiences. A body that receives higher source nutrients and continued caring maintenance will continue to thrive and maintain a high state of homoeostasis, meaning balanced health.

- It is vital that in order to *Navigate Life*, we need to take ownership of our health as the highest priority. In doing so, we de-accelerate the ageing process while our body remains healthy, vital and well.

- Many people hold an inaccurate belief that the body breaking down is part of the ageing process.

- Your body has a wisdom of its own. Given the correct environment, it knows what to do and how to do it.

- A person with a *Parked* mind set will generally entertain the same repeated thoughts and will not be conscious of their own thought pattern. They may be stuck in a repetitive feedback loop of toxic thoughts.

- Once your level of consciousness is raised we begin to impact our bodies in positive ways. Your thoughts influence your biology.

- While you may be *Navigating* in one area of your life, such as career, you may be stagnant and remain *Parked* in another area of your life such as relationships. This is not seen as bad, merely an opportunity to self-correct.

- Candace Pert wrote her book, *Molecules of Emotion*, about the body being the subconscious mind. Your body has a mind of its own.

- Approximately 80% of your immune system is contained within the gut. It is for this reason that what you eat and how you nourish your body relates to the health and well-being of your immune system.

- All body systems are inexorably linked and therefore cannot be isolated nor treated in isolation.

- View your body as a whole organic system, rather than attending to individual parts. Health and well-being become expressions of that way of thinking.

- To assist the body in its longevity, we must avoid certain toxic behaviors and habits that include excessive drinking, alcohol and drug abuse while maintaining a well-balanced and healthy lifestyle.

- *Navigating Life* in relation to your health and well-being, means that you are in conscious control of *how* and *what with* your body is nourished.

- People who are conscious and aware tend to choose foods that are in alignment with their highest potential.

- Knowing oneself becomes an essential component toward living a joyous, prosperous and healthy life.

- When we learn to live in tune with nature, we harness our genetic potential to activate our true genetic expression.

- The further we move away from nature in how we nourish our body and also through chronic exercise and stress, the less health and vitality we have in our later years.

- Your body knows and interprets every thought and emotion that takes place in your mind and body. There is no lying or no way that you can deceive your body with illegitimate thoughts.

- For a healthy body, any toxins or unhealthy food that is consumed will be quickly and effectively disposed of via one of the four detoxification organs of the body. A healthy, thriving cell will remove toxins immediately once they enter the cell.

- Your body is like a helium balloon, it is continually striving to maintain the highest state of homoeostasis and equilibrium.

- Obesity is not an intended function of Mother Nature's design. You need only look to the animal kingdom to see how effectively and effortlessly Mother Nature operates. It is rare to see animals living in the wild that are obese or overweight.

- Nature does not complicate what it can simplify.

- When you align yourself with the essential laws of healthy nutrition, your body will thrive and do so at the highest state of health and well-being with minimal effort.

Be open and receptive to listening to your body and being in tune to what your body is asking of you. Being receptive to these changes means having awareness toward nurturing your human form in another way.

CHAPTER SIX

A Health Perspective

Navigate Your Future Health. A Comparison

"If you don't take care of your body, where are you going to live?"

Unknown

	PARKED	NAVIGATING
DAILY	You find it hard to let go of the day's stress in order to unwind and rejuvenate.	You look forward to exercise and/or movement on a regular basis. You feel energized, alive post exercise.
WEEKLY	You are often in a stress-like state, which you are unable navigate your way out of.	Your body looks and feels young, with a sense of increased energy and vitality.
MONTHLY	Stress is now chronic. You gravitate toward drinking at night in order to relax and sleeping pills to help you sleep.	You have a well-defined physique with the right balance of muscle to fat.
YEARLY	Stress disrupts your health. You may be on the verge of developing an illness, having ignored the warning signs.	Your body composition and proportion rarely changes. You maintain good overall tone, muscle and immunity.

In the previous chapter we discussed the various levels of *Navigating Life* within the context of a health perspective. We looked at the four different levels and what it means to live at those various stages in relationship to our mental, emotional and physical well-being.

For many people who are in the early stages of their life, it may be difficult to look far into the future and imagine living well past eighty years of age. When young, we tend to live in the moment and give less regard to the future. .

In the table above you can see two columns *Parked* and *Navigating*. On the left-hand side of the table there are four chronological periods marked *Daily, Weekly, Monthly* and *Yearly*. Here we are looking at a state of health and viewing it from four perspectives. In the first box on the left-hand side you can see that we begin by looking at stress as a component of health.

The person who is *Parked* finds it difficult to let go of the day's stress in order to unwind and rejuvenate. Given the circumstances of this person's life, this may be a daily occurrence. This individual has a hard time letting go of stress whether the source is personal or professional. If we were to look at this person's weekly schedule, we would see that he is often in a stressed state and finds release difficult.

Fast forward two months' and we can see that the stress, which was once a daily occurrence, is now chronic. This individual may drink at night in order to relax or perhaps use sleeping pills in order to allow a deeper restful sleep. He still finds it challenging to turn off the stress cycle.

Finally, a year has lapsed and we can see that stress has now disrupted his health. He may be on the verge of developing an illness, having ignored the early warning signs which took place many months ago.

A cycle like the one presented above is all too common in our society today. An important consideration to understand is that repeated chronic stress can play havoc on physiological functions within the body. If left untreated, stress becomes a learned response, so much so that it inhibits and shuts down organ function as a means of preserving life. What we view as a disruption within the human ecosystem is in fact the human body preserving itself so that the chronic stress does not lead to a more debilitating condition.

The other chronic stress in our lives can also be exercise induced. Chronic Cardio may also be linked as a stress in so far as it activates the same fight or flight mechanism within the human brain. The mechanisms our bodies use to regulate stress are still quite similar to our ancestors who were chased by dangerous animals thousands of years ago.

The Cortisol Connection describes numerous scientific studies in which soldiers were tested to determine their stress levels at pre-and post-engagement in the field. Cortisol levels were taken prior to battle and then subsequently followed up upon their return from active duty. Many scientists had believed up to this point that once the body underwent chronic stress that it became inhibited and remained in this stress like state for a long time thereafter. These studies showed that although the soldier's cortisol levels had risen markedly during active engagement, upon returning home, in the majority of cases, cortisol levels returned to normal.

I have often heard people comment that they find it difficult and challenging to turn off at the end of the working day, given that their job may be highly stressful. In my experience, working one-on-one with corporate clients, I noted a common element in which many of the clients were "stuck" in a stress like state, It was almost as though the stress response had been jammed and every attempt to unlock the stress response, only seem to make things worse.

This goes back to the earlier point: if left unchecked chronic stress can become a habitual response which can overwhelm the mind and body.

The good news for many of us is that we have the ability to turn down the volume of repeated stress in our lives by becoming aware of our habitual patterns. If we examine the right hand side of the column where the individual is *Navigating Life*, we can see that this person looks forward to exercise and movement on a regular basis. They feel alive and energized through exercise and movement.

Looking forward, on a weekly basis we can see that the individual's body looks and feels young with a sense of increased energy and vitality. When this individual lives in accordance with their genetic blueprint, they activate the right type of physiological functions which are conducive toward sustaining and maintaining long-term health and vitality. They are not detracting, nor burdening the body through repeated chronic stress.

On a monthly basis this individual has a well-defined physique with the right ratio of muscle to fat. They tend to their physical regime in a manner that is not stressful, but rather promotes longevity and higher states of health. This person may undertake a combination of exercise and movement disciplines, which may range from resistance training, some light cardio, and perhaps a milder movement sequences to include yoga or Pilates.

Within a year this person's body composition and proportion rarely changes. They maintain good overall muscle tone, with the right immunity that is necessary for lasting health and well-being. It is essential that you strike a balance between the right type of exercises and movements in order to create the health and well-being your body needs to thrive on. If your day to day job entails continued stress and you find yourself wanting to run or lift heavy weights after work in order to release that stress, then you may be compounding the stress through your choice of vigorous exercise.

For some reason in our modern culture, we believe that more is better, when in fact more exercise may be responsible for tipping people over the edge. On many occasions when I have consulted with successful executives and CEO's, they are quite surprised to learn that I do not introduce exercise as part of their *Health and Well-being* program until at least three to five months into our work. My primary focus, in the initial stages of working one-on-one or in group situations, is to form healthy nutritional habits which allow the body to self-correct any physiological damage that may have been caused in the past due to these chronic stresses.

The initial phase normally involves the elimination of food toxins which may cause harm to the individuals mind and body. My purpose and aim is to get them out of this stress like state and into a parasympathetic state, thus allowing mind and body to be in homoeostasis. This can vary from person to person since different people respond accordingly to the external stimuli within their environment. We all have different thresholds of stress and it is important to never push oneself beyond those limits, since the long-term effects may be deleterious to the individual.

Self-awareness and self-examination becomes an important factor in order to become aware of habitual, chronic practices that allow the person to be exposed to repeated stress in their life. Far too many people re-live toxic and self-destructing behaviors because they are unconscious of these repeated patterns playing out in their life on an ongoing basis.

One must become aware of their unconscious thoughts, which manifest into conscious behavior. Self-awareness is a powerful vehicle for accessing and understanding the unconscious mind in this regard. We will examine this in further detail in the coming chapters, but now it is important that you understand the various dimensions of the mind and how they can influence your actions by drawing you closer toward health or further away into illness and disease.

When something relatively insignificant continually emerges in your life, but you do not have it in your conscious awareness, over time it can become a bigger problem that may lead to more complex health issues.

In order to Navigate your health, a simple and effective strategy, which can be used on a regular basis, is to "check-in" with yourself from time to time. Checking-in means acknowledging how you feel at the present moment in relationship to your health. Life is complex even at the best of times and we are managing various dimensions of our life, and most often on autopilot mode. Rarely do we stop to consider how we are actually performing in our life. This is critical because **life is not a dress rehearsal for a stage production – it is the stage production!** For this reason your life evolves and expands as you undergo many changes in cycles over time.

It is worthwhile checking in with yourself through self-examination, which is a powerful medium for delving in and examining your unconscious self. Before you recoil, thinking that this process is far too complex or that it requires a trained psychologist, be assured that all you are doing is posing questions to your subconscious mind in order to understand more about your true self.

A powerful question for opening up this dialogue with yourself may be as simple as asking yourself, *how am I doing* which is another way of asking, *how do I feel?* The question of how you feel allows you to pinpoint any emotional disturbances which may be going on at a deeper level. When you manage life from day to day, you seldom "check-in" to pose these questions.

The nature of self-examination is to avoid your health becoming *Parked.* For this exercise, you need to be as true and honest with your feelings before they avalanche into something greater. By this time it is generally too late, because when your emotions seek expression through your body, they will become stuck in an organ or a muscle. Therefore they inhibit or shutdown that body system so that you start to take notice and attend to these areas.

Remember that being *Parked* is not necessarily a bad thing. It merely denotes that you are in an undesirable state and that it is time to move out of this state and look at giving energy to any aspect of yourself which is either unconscious or not acknowledged. The wisdom of the human body is incredibly powerful. Your body is repeatedly talking to you and giving you feedback in relationship to your thoughts, beliefs, attitudes and emotions.

People who become chronically ill invariably have ignored the warning signs over time. These warning signs are messages from the body that relay information about your life and circumstances in order that you self-correct or adjust. For example you might be in friendship with someone who drains your energy as they unload their problems onto you. Since this is a close friend, one you do not want to offend you repeatedly listen to their problems, even though you become emotionally exhausted.

One of the symptoms that your body may offer is a headache after your meeting with your friend. You may dismiss this headache as simply being tired or dehydrated or anything else. It may not have occurred to you that your body is trying to tell you to distance yourself from this person.

Far too often this behavior can, seemingly go on for years before we realize that our friend was the cause of our headache and the ensuing health problems which manifested from that point on. In such instances it may be said that you are *Parked* because you fail to acknowledge and listen to the subtle cues that your body offers you in order to distance yourself from this friend. Your body is like a highly-intelligent tuning fork and receiver that takes in the information from its environment and processes it informing you if your encounters or interactions are conducive toward your health or detracting from it.

If we examine the opposite scenario we might see the person being inspired through their work by being of service. Your job or calling in life might be working with younger children. This could give you great joy to use your talents and skills to help those in need. When you are engaged in your work you find that is of a playful nature and time seems to stand still when you are doing what you love. You are inspired when you are working and this radiates through every cell of your body.

In this instance, you are following the guidance and becoming attuned to your environment. The very nature of your work is engaging and rewarding and that it communicates this message to every nerve and cell in your body, creating higher states of consciousness and also a higher state of *Health and Well-being.*

Finally *Navigating* your health means being attuned to the subtle changes and signs that your body continually offers you. On the other hand, people who neglect and ignore these signs can, if left unchecked, develop into something far more deadly.

You have the power, and now the resources, to create the health that you deserve in order to live a joyous, fulfilling and prosperous life, free of sickness and disease.

Chapter Summary

- Viewed from a perspective of *Parked* or *Navigating Life*, one can see that their immediate thoughts and perception create the health of tomorrow.

- I left untreated, stress may turn into a long term responses thereby inhibiting organ function and shutting down important biological functions within the body.

- Chronic cardio may be seen as a *stressor* to the body's ecological system when it is over prescribed. The body sees this as a fight or flight mechanism and thus rushes in to maintain equilibrium by suppressing organ function.

- Studies confirm that the human body is hard-wired to offset the demands of stress by returning to homeostasis once the stressor has been removed.

- Many people get stuck in a stressed state and find it challenging to let go of the day's stress, long after the event has taken place.

- The body may learn to become stuck in a stressed state and therefore shuts down major organ function in order to preserve life.

- If you work in a stressful job, be careful not to add to this through chronic exercise, which only adds to your body's inability to deal with the increased demand.

- When dealing with people whose jobs are stressful, attending to their nutritional requirements initially helps them reduce their stress levels significantly.

- The removal of toxins and poor lifestyle habits becomes paramount to reducing if not eliminating ones long term stress.

- Life is not a dress rehearsal for a stage production – it is the stage production!

- Use the checking-in method for examining ones unconscious thoughts.

- Simply asking oneself "how do I feel" is a good way to open up dialogue with yourself on a regular basis.

- The purpose of self-examination is to avoid becoming *Parked*.

- *Parked* is not necessarily a bad thing. It is life's way of providing your feedback so that you may *Navigate* your way back to safe ground again.

- Become attuned to your body's warning signs such as pain, feelings and sensations that are untoward. Your body is alerting you to something which is out of equilibrium.

- Your body is like a highly intelligent tuning fork, taking in information from your outside environment and processes internal. The result is a move toward health and wellbeing or chronic illness.

CHAPTER SEVEN
Navigate Life Wheel

Taking Inventory of Your Life

"The same wind blows on us all. The economic wind, the social wind, the political wind. The same wind blows on everybody. The difference in where you arrive in one year, three years, five years, the difference in arrival is not the blowing of the wind but the set of the sail."

Jim Rohn

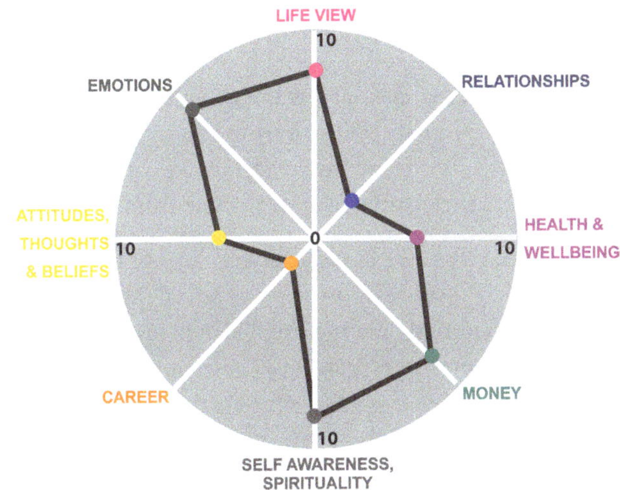

In the previous chapter we discussed the two elements of the health perspective. We looked at how life presents itself in relation to our health and well-being as seen from a *Navigating* perspective. In contrast, we examined the health perspective from a *Parked* viewpoint and saw that a person who is stagnant in relation to their health suffers over a long period of time as their health gradually deteriorates.

In this chapter we will examine the eight dimensions of *Navigating Life* and discuss how each of those dimensions work to influence one another. On the previous page, you can see the life wheel with eight different facets of life depicted by various colors. These various dimensions are:

- Life view
- Relationships
- Health and well-being
- Money
- Self-awareness and spirituality
- Career
- Attitude, thoughts and beliefs
- Emotions

Each aspect of the eight dimensions has the potential to influence the other. When you are aware that you are managing these eight dimensions, or houses, you are empowered to make conscious decisions based on how you are performing in each of these areas.

Starting from the middle of the circle, and working our way out to the edge of the circle, the life wheel is given a numerical rating ranging from 0 up to 10. The numbers 0 to 5 are represented as being *Parked*, while the numbers 5 to 10 represents *Navigating Life* within that dimension. As we discussed in previous chapters, being *Parked* is not necessarily an undesirable state. It merely gives you an indication of how you are performing within this particular dimension. It is wise to take stock of your life on a regular basis.

Let us analyse this via the use of an example that clearly demonstrate how each of the eight aspects work together to allow you to successfully *Navigate Life*. If your life is low, ranging between zero and five, this has the potential to impact other aspects of your life.

If you refer back to the previous chapters, where we discussed the qualities of a *Parked* state in relation to the life view, you might recall a person's outlook on life when in a *Parked* state is stagnant and not moving forward when compared with a *Navigating* state. This *life view* has the potential to influence and affect other aspects of the life wheel. If one's mental outlook is of negativity, then it stands to reason that the way this person responds to life may also be of a similar nature.

Your *life view* is the strongest aspect of the eight dimensions, and influences the other eight dimensions since it is a strong component of your overall consciousness level. A person who is *Navigating Life* tends to hold a strong *life view* which incorporates higher states of mental thought. Your predominant thoughts affect and influences your emotional well-being. What you hold in mind as your recurring thoughts are brought about in your reality.

If your *life view* is one of a *Parked* state then this has the capacity to influence other areas of your life wheel. A person who is *Parked* in their *life view* will generally have attitudes which limit in nature. Rather than seeing opportunities present themselves in life, their tendency will be orientated toward problems since they are resonating at a lower frequency. This is not conducive toward viewing a reality from a different viewpoint.

A person who is in a high *Navigating* state with respect to their career may simultaneously have a low *Parked* state within their relationship house. It might be that in order to bring home the money and live a certain quality of life, they work long hours, which has an impact on your romantic relationship with your husband or wife. Each aspect of our lives has the potential to influence and affect other aspects of our lives. The key in any of the areas is to be aware of what is happening in one's life at any given point and to take action in order to circumvent any negative result.

Often enough, people orientate themselves toward a handful of these dimensions at the risk of neglecting some of the others. What you value and hold dear to you is where your attention and focus will be given. For example, if you value relationships and health more than money or career, then this will be a much higher rating than the other two areas. Now this does not mean that you are lacking in the other two areas, it may simply give you some feedback as to how you are performing in the area of the money and career.

Life is a process of evolving and growing. It is important you understand this, in that any result that you begin to see showing up in your life, is in effect as a result of the attention or energy that is being directed toward that area. If you value money or career, then the life you live offers you the ability to chart a new course and give more attention and focus to that area in order to create the reality that you wish to see.

Navigating Life is a perpetual journey, ever evolving and changing, which entails making mistakes along the way. Hopefully you learn from your mistakes and do not repeat them as you continue to *Navigate Life*. You are the product of each area that you repeatedly draw your attention toward. The more attention and energy that is given to that area, the more likely it is you will be able to experience breakthroughs and success in life.

It is important that you do not get stuck in a negative state when life offers you a negative experience. This may show up from time to time and it is important to understand that sometimes situations in your life are being worked out, and in doing so, something needs to give in order to make way for the new element to emerge. Become alert to staying fixed on certain outcomes—do not get invested in thinking that life needs to serve you or owes you anything because you are a good person or are doing it tough. This is incorrect thinking and should be examined as soon as you become aware of it.

Let us examine the eight dimensions in more detail while paying close attention to the qualities of each house and how they relate to your overall state of *Navigating Life*.

Life View

Your *life view* may be defined as your overall outlook on life expressed through your values and beliefs. Your beliefs have a powerful effect on your general outlook on life since they influence your perception. Your perception can be understood as the filter in which you perceive your reality.

Your *life view* may be influenced through personal experience insofar as it is an accumulation of your thoughts, words, actions and experiences up until this point in your life. Therefore, your current view of reality is shaped and influenced by your past.

For example, maybe you have heard people out of a newly dissolved romantic relationship declare the probability high of future romantic relationships being the same as in the past. The human brain is clever in anticipating and determining future events by looking back on historical or past events as a guide. It is believed that we rarely think any new thoughts on a daily basis. Much of our thought patterns, (approximately 70,000 thoughts a day) mainly consist of repetitive thoughts.

Your mind is attuned to making future predictions based on the past experiences. Your mind also uses your values and beliefs about the world as the brush from which to paint your future canvas. It is for this reason that many people find it challenging to break habitual patterns that have been ingrained in their neural network for many years.

Your belief about reality influences the likelihood of your future arriving in such a way. Let us examine a simple example, such as finding a car space within a busy city location. I have often heard people recount stories about how they can never find a car space when they drive into the city. The same has also been true of those who have spoken about the ease and simplicity at being able to find a car space within the same location. Whilst this represents a simple version of how a belief can play out in one's life, it nonetheless demonstrates the power of beliefs to shape your reality.

In relation to the *Navigating* model, we want to create empowering beliefs which are neither shaped nor influenced by our past beliefs or childhood programs. Our childhood programs may be viewed as a set of instructions and directives that were given to us by respected and valued authority at a young age. It is believed that most of our beliefs are formed between the ages of two and seven. Subsequently, many of these beliefs may be challenged and examined at the age of nine or ten as the young adolescent mind begins to formulate his or her own opinions about their world.

How *do* we create empowering beliefs when our past circumstances or reality has shown us otherwise? It is important to see our beliefs in a new context by regularly examining their validity. To put it simply, in order for the brain to function optimally, the software downloaded needs to be examined and updated to express the new view of reality.

In order to change your future, it is important to change the inner dialogue and programming which largely influences your view of reality. You have no doubt been exposed to situations in your own life where your repeated behavior was not congruent with the life you desired. For example, it may be your desire to lose weight, yet you snack on food which is not conducive toward maintaining health and well-being. If so, then it might be prudent to examine any unconscious beliefs that are holding you back from achieving your desired results.

There may be self-sabotaging beliefs that thwart your intentions to create and maintain long-term health. Awareness is a powerful tool for recognizing self-deprecating behavior which allows us to adjust our course in order to create a better version of reality. Life offers us the opportunity to self-correct our situation by offering us the chance to become aware of our predominant thought patterns. This is the greatest offering that life has given you: the ability to chart your destiny anew each day.

In order to have a *life view* that represents your wants and desires, it is essential that you become aware and reframe your core beliefs about reality. Albert Einstein said, *you cannot solve a problem with the same level of thinking that created it*. Therefore, if whatever is showing up in your life is not an aspect that you wish to see, you must change the level of thinking and create a new mind from which to create your future. Your mind and your thinking shape and augment your reality, since what you think about you draw into your reality.

Not surprisingly, continual self-examination can in some instances be arduous. It is not my intention to dissuade you, though it is practical and worthwhile to mention that self-development is a continual process of refinement and subtle changes that evidently give way to greater results.

Life is not merely a cause and effect reality as many people are led to believe. You may have heard someone use the expression, *I'll give it a go and see what transpires*. This mode of thinking is dependent on a cause and effect model. If you give it a go, the situation might work out, yet there is also the probability that it will work against you.

The purpose of developing a stronger and more powerful life that is congruent with your deepest desires, is that **you become inspired to create the outcome you wish to see take place in your life**. If it is your desire to be a successful writer and you attend a number of short writing courses with the view of writing a novel and ultimately being published, then nothing will stop you from achieving that reality. It is almost certain that you will be faced with challenges, setbacks and obstacles along the path of your desire. These challenges are not meant to stop you, nor to dissuade you from becoming a successful writer, rather the challenges are offering you the opportunity for self-grow in order to give you the tools and resources you will need when you become a successful writer.

You cannot become successful, whilst entertaining lower states of consciousness. You must transcend your current level of thinking to higher dimensions in order to gain the success you wish to realize.

Your *life view* is your preview into your destiny. In order to shape your destiny, you must be supported by empowering and positive beliefs which align with your proposed future. It is for these reasons that *Navigate Life* sets out to enrich you with valuable tools and resources to assist you in becoming the person required to fulfill your purpose and destiny.

Let us now examine point number two of the *Life Wheel* by looking at a detailed approach to relationships.

Relationships encompass, not only intimate and romantic relationships, but also those relationships that embody the context of your life. Such relationships may be the one you have with family, with friends, with work colleagues or other types of relationships in your life.

Relationships

Your relationships are an integral aspect of your being. Your relationships with others are a barometer of your self worth. You have no doubt heard the saying that relationships are a mirror of our deepest selves. Most people link the word *relationships* to intimacy. As we have discussed earlier - romantic relationships represent one aspect of the total relationship you have with self.

The majority of problems one faces in life can be attributed to three main areas: health, finance and relationships. It is apparent that managing these life areas is taxing and complex given the volatility that each aspect encompasses. I use the word volatility to define the improbable nature in which our health, finances and relationships fluctuate.

We discussed in the earlier point of *life view* that our most predominant beliefs are responsible for the reality we create. Relationships are an extension of our *life view* beliefs since many of our thoughts and ideas about what constitutes healthy relationships are generally formed from a young age.

Psychologists believe that this attachment style is generally formed between the ages of zero and six years of age. Almost 70 to 80% of adult behavior reflects this attachment style developed in early life. Therefore, the nurturing you received as a child from parents or guardians is influential to the way in which you form relationships as an adult.

We all want to have fulfilling and lasting relationships, whether they are of an intimate, professional, familial or friendship. When relationships go sour, they not only impact the other party or parties involved, they also reflect back on you, thus causing a myriad of emotional disturbances. Remember, that you are repeatedly creating and maintaining relationships with others and yourself.

Your success in forming empowering relationships hinges on the relationship you have with yourself. Your self-worth and self-esteem is indicative of the manner in which people reflect to you what you believe about yourself. Moreover, is not uncommon to see someone of low self-esteem form intimate relationships with those of high self-esteem. The concern with this behavior underlies the mechanism in which intimate relationships dissolve since there is an unmatched level of power within the relationship. I am not suggesting that relationships should be orientated toward a power play; rather there should be an equal distribution of energy between two people that lead to fulfilling and harmonious relationships. Certainly at periods throughout the relationship, the allocation or distribution of power may be one-sided, although I believe that nature is far more intelligent and there is a deeper understanding that one needs to learn during these moments in life. The underlying lesson may be a call for leadership in order to sustain the relationship and create a harmonious outcome.

As part of your relationship journey, there are times when you will Navigate within the context of a relationship. If you recall earlier in the book, we mentioned the *Navigating* and *Parked* roadmap, which consisted of an infinity symbol with the left colored red representing *Parked*, whilst the right was colored green, representing Navigation.

From this understanding, if you apply the context of your relationships in your life as being either *Parked* or *Navigating*, it will allow you the opportunity to attend to those relationships which may be in the *Parked* category. The purpose of the tools contained within the book is to give you awareness and a roadmap toward creating successful outcomes throughout your life. Pain and suffering occurs when we are unconscious or unaware of our repeated habits and patterns that seemingly creep up on us, and if left unchecked may eventually cause irreconcilable repair.

Toward the end of this book you will find a *Navigating* and *Parked* questionnaire which allows you to examine each of the eight dimensions contained within this chapter. Whilst it may be challenging to be 100% in each of the dimensions, it provides an opportunity for you to check-in through regular self-examination and make adjustments where necessary.

The purpose of life is not necessarily to get somewhere in any length of time. Life is a continual process of learning, acquiring new understandings, resources and tools that allow you to master the process of life. It is inevitable that giving your best effort to attend to each of these eight dimensions, you will undoubtedly be met with challenges, disappointments and heartache along the journey. Do not be discouraged nor dissuaded from learning or acquiring new understanding and inner wisdom. For even during those moments of despair, when it seems like all your best intentions have been thwarted, particularly in your relationships, it is at these times that your greatest growth will occur.

You, yourself, are the measure that dictates the way in which people will react to you and treat you. Your self-worth and self-esteem is either the beacon that will direct those safely toward you or signal them away. We show others how we wish to be treated. Those who are involved in intimate relationships and suffer low self-esteem may be less adept at standing up for their self-worth. This results in the other party taking advantage of the relationship by dominating through their self-worth.

From an outside perspective, others might look at this relationship as toxic or destructive, where in fact the relationship may be deemed harmonious within its own context. The harmony of the relationship continues since where there is low self-worth in one of the partners, then there is an opposing force taking control of the relationship. Relationships have a dynamic interplay that allow for adjustments and calibration, until the time this harmonious union can no longer exist. At this point there is either dissolution of the relationship or tension emerges in order to bring the relationship back into harmony.

To recap: Your relationship with others is a reflection of the relationship you hold with yourself. What you believe and think about yourself, at the deepest level, is what others will be drawn to or opposed to.

Your connection with others provides the framework to validate these thoughts and beliefs. Others are only reflecting back what you know to be true of yourself. It is for this reason that relationships should not be viewed as challenging or difficult, rather as an opportunity to look inward in an attempt to improve the inner landscape. Like a flourishing garden, the more you tend to your weeds, by pulling them out as they arise, the more beautiful the garden will flourish with time. The key is to tend to the aspects of oneself which have mirrored back to you via your relationships.

Certainly, it can be disheartening at times when your friend or co-worker accuses you of something you disregard yourself to be. Yet it also provides an opportunity to heal this aspect of your nature so that it falls away and does not become a dominating component of who you really are. You are more than your beliefs and thoughts about yourself. These are merely stories that you created at a point in time to conceal the inner beauty of the real you from emerging. I believe it is vital that we return back to our authentic nature, which is the pure awareness of consciousness. Anything else you believe yourself to be or not to be is merely a facade, one that keeps you imprisoned in an unauthentic body.

Your relationships with others influence other aspects of the *Life Wheel* and it is vital that you become orientated toward creating health and lasting relationships throughout your life.

Health and Well-being

In previous chapters we examined the context of what health and well-being encompasses and the qualities that are apparent when you are *Navigating* your health. Within the context of the *Life Wheel*, health and well-being is one of the eight dimensions which influence the other houses.

In this section we look at how your health influences and affects other aspects of your Life View.

We previously identified that your overall state of well-being is a springboard toward living a fulfilling and prosperous life. In the earlier chapters, we saw that one's state of health creates a lever toward personal power. Your personal power is that element that defines you as you *Navigate Life* equipping you with the tools and resources to live an abundant and successful life. Sure people might wince and suggest that their grandfather or great aunt lived to ninety-four years of age and was a packet a day smoker. Genetic research is showing us that despite "bad habits" such as smoking, a small portion of the population are relatively unaffected. For the majority though, our genes have the potential to express disease or illness, which may be inherited through generations.

Epigenetics reminds us that our environment has a greater influence on gene expression that the genes we inherit. In other words, genes may be turned "on" or "off" depending on lifestyle choices. In the book, *Pottenger's Prophecy*, the authors state that 70% of illness and disease can be prevented through better lifestyle choices. They go on to cite the work of pediatrician Dr. Alan Greene, saying that every bite you eat is an investment in your future, or it is a debt you are taking out. So make sure you are investing wisely when you go to the grocery store.

The power to control and influence your health destiny, as the author states, is largely at the control of your volition. This is great news since people believed in previous decades that their default genes were the determining factor in their state of health and wellbeing. Science now tells us that we have a 70% chance of preventing illness through better lifestyle choices.

While this information may be a relief for many people, the downside is that we still need to do the work in order to stave off disease and the associated risks that come with living in a modern world. We are all moving toward death from the moment we are born. The choices we make and the thoughts we regularly entertain, determine the rate at which we arrive at our last breath. The good news is that it does not have to be that way and despite the consensus that living a healthy lifestyle is challenging, it need not be that way if people start slowly and advance slowly in the direction of healthy lifestyle choices.

The *Life Wheel* diagram is interconnected and so what you experience in one area or dimension has the potential to affect other areas of your overall *Life Wheel*. Imagine having low energy, continually sick, and despondent about life. How do you imagine life would look in comparison to someone who maintains a healthy and vibrant outlook?

Now you might interrupt me at this point stating that a decline in health is inevitable as we age. Yes, that may be the case if you have made poor health choices during the course of your earlier life. The wisdom of the body catches up to you eventually. You cannot expect to run your body like a motor vehicle and expect it to perform like a Ferrari.

Your body is a dynamic organism which is forever seeking the highest expression of health. It is our poor habits and lifestyle choices that thwart the body's ability to maintain a level of homeostasis. Getting back to the earlier example of having low energy and fatigue, this has a far rippling effect on your overall Life View, insofar as your choices become limited in what you are able to achieve and perform. Imagine for a moment that you wake up one day tired, even though you had nine hours of restful sleep. You still feel groggy and your head and thoughts feel heavy and lucid. As the morning and day progresses, you find it difficult to shake that feeling from your head. Everything seems like a slow dream sequence unfolding before your eyes.

It is an hour later after you have just woken up and you need another nap. You comfortably fall asleep and later wake up only to realize that hours have passed. That groggy feeling is still apparent and you are still unmotivated and unenthusiastic about venturing outside to get some sunlight. You would rather stay indoors, and better yet, stay in bed for the remainder of the day.

Oddly enough, this scenario is far too common in many people's lives. Those who have suffered chronic depression or adrenal fatigue know all too well how limiting life can be when their health has been compromised. They yearn for the simplest of things, such as playing with their children or taking the dog for a walk.

We are born with energy and vitality, and depending on how we spend that energy during our lifetime, it either accumulates in our later years or diminishes, leaving us apathetic and unenthusiastic toward life. I am sure you know of people who fit this category all too well—the ones who are forever complaining how tough life is and complain that there is not enough time and energy to do the things they used to do. They reminisce about the past and feel that ageing is to blame for their current life situation.

On the other hand I like to remind these same people, that there are others who have made wise and healthy choices toward maintaining and enhancing their well-being, who are living rich and rewarding lives. What you give is what you get back. Where you choose to invest your time and energy is how life rewards you in the future.

Money

Your relationship with money stems from your predominant beliefs about money. These relationships are held at the level of the subconscious mind and influence the way in which money comes into our life with ease and perfection or equally disappears from our hands in the same manner.

For those who live from paycheck to paycheck, barely making ends meets and struggling to save enough money, the truth of the matter lies within a deep-seated belief system which stops the flow of money entering their life. Money is an energy system that is attracted to or repelled according to one's predominant thoughts about money and themselves.

It is my belief that society and our schooling system do not give enough value toward the creation of wealth and also the management of money. We learn to manage money as a result of the familial influences that are acquired from a young age. You may have grown up in a family situation where the phrases "money doesn't grow on trees" and "money is the root of all evil" were repeated by loved ones or parents.

My personal situation was that I grew up in a family of working class, migrant parents who came to this country with little financial resource. It was through sheer hard work and diligent saving that they were able to afford the luxuries that most people nowadays take for granted.

I recall as a young child asking my father for a bicycle and hearing the words, *Money doesn't grow on trees!* as one of his regular mantras. His understanding was that a bicycle was not a necessity, rather more of a luxury. With two other siblings to care of, it was not of great importance that we spend money on a new bicycle.

It was only through determination and hard work that I eventually took on a paper delivery run that afforded me the luxury of riding a bicycle so as to deliver newspapers. This also allowed me to develop a sound relationship with money. In retrospect, not having enough money was possibly one of the strongest groundings, since it taught me to value money in a unique way.

At the time it was difficult to comprehend why other children my age were given a bicycle for their birthdays or Christmas, whereas, I had to work for my bicycle. This gave me a tremendous security and appreciation for money.

Your relationship with money has the potential to affect and influence the other seven dimensions within your life wheel. Think about those moments throughout your life when money was scarce? How did you feel at the time? How did the lack of money influence your self-esteem?

When money is scarce, there is a direct correlation to self-esteem. You need only look at rich and successful businessman and note the level of confidence and high self-esteem they hold. Consequently, those who have a scarcity mindset to money are also affected by other factors within their life wheel.

Having a scarcity mindset might detract from pursuing a career of your interest. For example you might undertake a non-rewarding job only to meet your financial commitments. In such a case, your self-esteem takes a direct hit since you feel there is never enough money to go around.

Navigating Life seeks to arm you with the mental resources to develop a prosperity and abundance mindset by honoring your self-worth. When you are *Navigating* your finances, money flows into your life with ease and perfection. You choose to pursue your purpose in life rather than performing at a job. By doing so, you honor yourself by expressing your unique talents and gifts and thus revealing them to the world. In recognition, the universe acknowledges your gifts and talents as an expression of your deepest self. Money will speedily flow into your life when you align yourself with this truth.

For many people, there are the limiting beliefs which emerge based around the concept of self-worth and money. The internal conversations that play out in one's mind may be, *who would want to pay me for this service or I could never make enough money and sustain a successful life doing what I love.*

I speak from experience with respect to this internal dialogue, as there were a number of limiting beliefs that emerged in my adult life as an expression of the predominant beliefs I picked up as a child. When I eventually started working for myself, I initially found it challenging and frightening. Instead of relying on a weekly paycheck, I now had to go out and look for clients in order to draw a weekly income. This was daunting at first since I was also facing the frightening aspect of subsequently dealing with my limiting beliefs about money. It was only when I faced these beliefs head-on through regular self-examination, that I was able to see the underlying emotion that was attached to my relationship with money.

Fear and anxiety are generally the two emotions which influence your ability to attract money into your life. Fear informs us of many contradictory beliefs about money that generally start with the phrase, *what if?*" For a moment think about your relationship with money and the emotion that emerges when you entertain a scarcity mindset? For example you might check your bank accounts one day only to discover that the balance is far lower than you anticipated. You check your calendar only to realize there are upcoming bills and expenses that need to be met and in no time your thoughts begin to race about the impending doom, fretting about money and now oscillating between fear and anxiety.

Given that we spoke about the universal law which states that *like attracts like*, how possible is it that money is likely to easily flow into your life considering your destructive thought patterns at this stage?

Self-Awareness and Spirituality

One of the significance aspects of *Navigate Life* is the *self-awareness* and *spiritual* principles, which in conjunction with the other foundational elements creates an all-encompassing program that helps you take control and ownership of your life.

As we have previously examined, *Self-awareness* embodies the principles of knowing oneself at a deeper core level. The basis to *Navigating Life* is rooted in the understanding and knowledge of oneself. The Greek philosopher Socrates said, know thyself. Self-knowledge is vested in self-empowerment, which is the basis for *Navigating Life* rather than being stagnant or *Parked.* I believe that a great deal of mankind's problems are infused in the lack of understanding that each have of themselves. To truly know and understand oneself at a deeper level means to acknowledge the duality of your nature. Life becomes a dance as you unify and acknowledge that you are a multi-dimensional being capable of achieving so much.

When you are self-aware you make decisions that are congruent with the deepest aspect of yourself. Your life choices become an extension of your deepest wants and desires since these are aspects of your authentic self. In contrast those who remain *Parked* respond to life by not taking charge of their own life. They may have little self-knowledge about their wants and needs and this may be reflected in their poor life choices. These life choices are mirrored in the eight dimensions within the life wheel.

The purpose of this chapter is to explain how each of these eight dimensions affects and influences the other dimensions. If we were to remove one or two of these dimensions, they would affect the overall success of being able to *Navigate Life.*

By being self-aware you are able to make choices that mirror your deepest desires. In doing so you create better life choices that resonate with your authentic self.

There is a great deal of talk nowadays about the pursuit of happiness. Scientists, philosophers and spiritual advocates have all thrown their hat into the ring stating their perspective on how to attain happiness. My belief is that happiness becomes an extension of being truly aligned and congruent with one's authentic self.

Your authentic self is the spiritual essence of who you are. It is the embodiment of your qualities, your gifts, your talents and that aspect of your inner light which others are aware of.

Self-awareness and *spirituality* work in harmony and unison with one another, they are one relationship, coexisting together. Spirituality calls for the understanding that you are not just a human being comprised of flesh and bone. You are a multi-dimensional, spiritual being that is an expression of universal intelligence. You have the genetic coding that is more intelligent than you can ever comprehend.

Spirituality seeks to understand that you are not here on this earth merely to exist, consume and then die. You have a reason and purpose for being a part of this universal cosmos and when you begin to understand and acknowledge this, your true self begins to emerge. Your talents and gifts are unique to you since no other person on this planet embodies these qualities in the same manner that you do. Your greatest realization and obstacle is to accept the enormity of this statement and seek to encapsulate the essence of who you are by expressing these qualities.

Despite today's misconceptions about spiritual people being tree-hugging hippies who subsist on vegetarian food, it is pleasing to know that some of the world's most notable and successful people are, in fact, spiritual in nature. One of the most prominent spiritual hippies of our time was none other than the late founder and CEO of Apple computers, Steve Jobs. Steve had a strong connection with Zen Buddhism which shaped and influenced a large aspect of the creativity that he brought forward to his work at Apple.

It is worth noting the difference between spirituality and organized religion since it appears that for most people the two are connected. Organized religion dictates a way of being that is governed by doctrines and practices established to guide their followers. For example, the Catholic Church stipulates the following of the Ten Commandments, decreeing a code of conduct that Catholics must abide by. *Thou shalt not commit adultery* and *Thou shalt keep holy the Sabbath* are examples of commandments dictated by the church. Judaism dictates seven laws that include: Prohibition of Idolatry, Prohibition of Murder, Prohibition of Theft, Prohibition of Sexual Promiscuity, and Prohibition of Blasphemy, Not to eat the flesh of an animal while it is alive. The requirement to have just Laws and government to police the preceding six laws.

Spirituality on the other hand is not grounded in law and established practices. Spirituality affirms, unlike organized religion, that there are many paths to God. This is echoed in the saying, *There are many paths to the top of the mountain, but the view is all the same.* Spirituality defines human beings as all connected through a sense of oneness. Your thoughts and actions influence and affect each other, and based on this principle, it is befitting that we all operate from the same principle of oneness and love as the basis to universal connection.

The understanding is that your belief in a greater intelligence influences your outlook and life view. You are more prone to take a universal view of creation and the universe, rather than an individualistic view that stipulates there is nothing after I die and I am here for a short period of time, so I should make the most of it. This is a limited way of thinking since it neglects to acknowledge that there could be a greater force operating in the universe.

Self-awareness and *spirituality* work synergistically with the other dimensions in an integrated manner to allow a unified and integrated union of the *Navigating Life* principles. One is not complete without the other and it is essential that one integrates the various principles into their life consistently and slowly over time.

It is important to understand and appreciate the fundamental components of *self-awareness* and *spirituality* that are aligned with a universal outlook.

Career

Your career is an important and valuable component of your *Navigating Life*. Your career works simultaneously and in harmony with the other seven dimensions to bring about an integrated life view. I am sure you have been in a situation where you have experienced familial or intimate relationship issues that found their way into your work life. Despite your best intentions to compartmentalize each component of your life and restrict them crossing over, the reality is that this is not as straightforward as one would hope.

To create a successful career you should look to balance the other seven dimensions within your life view. If you have ever read biographies or books on successful leaders, you may have noted how seemingly balanced every aspect of their life is. This is not coincidental but purposely orchestrated so that other dimensions of their life do not affect their career. Successful leaders treat their career as a sport insofar as their dedication and commitment toward their career is 100%.

To have a successful and rewarding career in whatever field or industry you work in, relies on maintaining balance and *Navigating Life* within the other seven dimensions. The beauty of *Navigating Life* is that it offers you the ability to look at life as a dashboard, where all the gages are within your view and the ability to adjust is within your reach.

As you have noticed in the previous pages with the *Life Wheel*, there is a rating between zero and ten that I suggest you routinely examined and complete so that you have a working understanding of where you sit within that continuum.

Routinely checking in affords you the opportunity to paying attention to any area that requires your attention and energy. As humans we can be very driven and focused in a number of life pursuits, to the detriment of others slipping out of our hands. For example your relationships and your health can affect your career in many ways. For this reason, what takes place in your relationships, whether they are of an intimate nature, business or friends can have a long-standing impact on your emotional well-being. Your emotional well-being is an important driver for your performance level within your career. Concurrently, the state of your health also impacts on your career since it can be the jewel performance of work on a day-to-day basis.

In my one-on-one work with professional clients and within corporate environments, I treat every individual as though they were an athlete. The definition of the athlete is anyone that performs at the highest level in order to produce a result or an outcome. Many executive's, CEOs and leaders of companies fit this description perfectly since not only do they have to perform at the highest level, they also need to manage, inspire and motivate people within their organization. It is paramount that they tend to their health, their relationships and the other components of the *Navigate Life* regularly in order to operate at the highest level.

So we can see that performance within one's career is directly related to and influenced by other *Navigating Life* dimensions. You may consider your thoughts in each of the eight dimensions and that your focus may deviate or change depending on your life situation. Given this analogy, you are managing eight different dimensions which require that you bring eight different managerial and leadership qualities to each of those dimensions.

Undoubtedly, along the way you will encounter problems and challenges in managing those eight respective areas. Do not be discouraged or disheartened if situations slide, since in this model of *Navigating* versus *Parked*, there are no mistakes, only opportunities to rectify and improve upon a current state.

If you refer to the *Life View* as given earlier, you can see that career sits opposite *relationships*. The purpose of this is to highlight the importance of your relationships as a means of support within your career. It is worth acknowledging that if you have successful and fulfilling relationships, then it is likely that you will have a successful career given the support mechanism. On the other hand, if your relationships are struggling and unhealthy, there is a high incidence that your career will also reflect these challenges.

I would like you to take away from this chapter the understanding and importance of the life wheel working as an encompassing component of your life. Understanding and appreciating that all eight dimensions support and complements one another while simultaneously working independent of each other. We could have easily used a square or rectangle to demonstrate the various eight dimensions, although I feel that tends to compartmentalize each component without giving weight to the relationship of each working independently and yet as a whole.

Wherever you stand at present in your career, whether it is a junior role, middle management, senior management or leadership role within the company, learn to appreciate the dynamics of each component of the *Life Wheel* by regularly checking and examining where you are placed within those dimensions. In previous chapters I talked about the importance of regularly checking in by asking the question, *how do I feel?* This allows you to attend to any impending situations before they arise.

Attitude, Thoughts and Beliefs

The seventh dimension is appropriately listed as your *Attitudes, Thoughts and Beliefs.* I have purposely combined all these three elements together since I believe they work in harmony and in unison as a cohesive group.

Let us break them down into each component by examining how each relate to one another, whilst also working independently and in collaboration with the other dimensions of *Navigating Life.*

Attitude

Your *Attitude* is your gauge and barometer toward life. Your attitude can thwart your success or can prepare you for amazing heights. Your attitude is your driving force, and the engine that propels you forward in life. It is the manner in which you respond to life and the lenses in which you choose to view your circumstances.

Without doubt the people who successfully *Navigate Life* and create their own circumstances have a positive mindset and attitude which is reflected by how life simultaneously is reflected back to them. Conversely, those who regularly entertain negative thoughts and have a low or pessimistic outlook on life, seemingly attract those same circumstances into their life.

Jim Rohn, the famous motivational speaker said, *the same wind blows on us all; the difference is the set of sail.* We all have a cross to bear in life and our challenges vary by degrees, but all the same. As Rohn reminds us, it is how we set our sail that determines our course and journey throughout life.

Attitude is an acquired characteristic that is either positive or negative based on your interpretation of events that have taken place throughout your life. You have no doubt heard inspirational stories about people who have overcome challenges and setbacks in their life, having developed a positive attitude towards life. They used their setbacks to inspire and motivate, rather than be defeated by them.

Your attitude is your response to life, and optimists would have you know that when life throws you lemons, you better make lemonade. What this really tells us is that your journey in life is bound to be met with obstacles and challenges and rather than allow these hurdles to taint your perception of life, you should take what you are given and create the ideal circumstances to give purpose and meaning to your life.

In the coming chapters we will examine a blueprint for taking charge of your life by empowering you with positive thoughts and beliefs.

Thoughts

We process anywhere between 60,000 to 70,000 thoughts a day. Many of these thoughts are on a feedback loop, meaning that we have entertained these thoughts repeatedly in previous days and weeks. Reflect on this for a moment. When was the last time you had an original thought? An original thought might be viewed as an idea or an inspirational thought rather than the habitual thoughts which you process day to day.

You might be surprised to learn that it may be days or weeks since your last original thought. When I tried this exercise, my most recent original thought occurred three days ago. I was alarmed to learn, like many other people that our predominant thought patterns are in fact of repetitive nature.

Since we process so many thoughts a day it becomes increasingly difficult to filter out what is relevant to our lives and what we should discard. I have often spoken to busy corporate executives who have trouble getting to sleep each night as a result of their frantic thought patterns. They are attempting to live in the past, in the presence and the future simultaneously, whilst trying to maintain a normal life. It is no wonder that many of them are plagued with anxiety and high levels of stress, since they are either stuck in the past or looking toward an anticipated future.

Dan Millman in his book, *Way of the Peaceful Warrior*, presents a simple yet profound concept—**the time is now, the place is here**. Stay in the present. You can do nothing to change the past, and the future will never come exactly as you plan or hope for." Therefore, all that we have is contained within the present moment. We will look at this concept more deeply in the coming chapters as we devote an entire section on learning to live in the present moment.

Sometimes it feels like our thoughts are hurtling out of control like a car on an icy road. Whilst our best intentions are to stay on the road and avoid crashing, we undoubtedly focus on the brick wall ahead and soon enough we can no longer tolerate these incessant thoughts. It is at this point that our stress levels exceed our healthy level and in no time our mind and body shuts down in order to preserve life.

If you are lucky enough to heed the warning signals, then you will most likely take immediate action to avoid crashing down. Sadly enough, most people take the opposite approach and put their foot down on the accelerator by choosing substances, such as caffeine and alcohol to maintain their level of awareness and energy levels. Your thoughts influence your physiology and this is no more evident than when you receive bad news and your heart beat begins to dramatically rise. In no time soon you may become anxious and develop an ill feeling in your stomach.

This is a process which happens many times a day for most people, before they get "stuck" in this loop pattern and they have taught their body to be stressed. The good news is that it does not have to be this way. You have the power to tame your thoughts by not repeatedly responding to them and giving them energy. In the coming chapters we shall look at some ways that you can take ownership of your thoughts by not being invested in them.

For now it is important to understand that your thoughts are comprised of a system that determines whether you stay *Parked* or *Navigate Life*.

Beliefs

We discussed in some detail how beliefs shape our perception of reality, so now let us look at how beliefs work together with our thoughts and attitude as a way of *Navigating Life*.

If you have a strong belief toward goodness and success in life, your subconscious thoughts are orientated to look for evidence in your life to support this belief. Previously, we discussed the idea of looking for a car park and having the affirmative belief that you will find a car park when you set out to drive into the city. I reference this example by citing my mother who worries about not being able to find a car park when she drives into the CBD. On the other hand, I hold an empowering belief toward finding a suitable car park each and every time I drive into the city.

Neither of us is right or wrong, it just turns out that we have developed a different set of beliefs based on past conditioning, experiences and circumstances. Undoubtedly we have used these past circumstances to create and shape our future reality. Your beliefs have the potential to shape your reality in a positive or negative way.

To successfully *Navigate Life* it is important that you create and examine your beliefs on a repeated basis to determine whether they are working in your favor. If the belief does not empower you to manifest the reality that you desire, then you should either examine the validity of that belief or drop the belief altogether.

It makes sense that in many instances our beliefs have been formed over many years and are rarely examined. This is because they are held within the unconscious mind and to examine them requires your conscious attention. It is for this reason that many people forego this process believing that it is arduous and time-consuming. When you are successfully *Navigating Life* you will undoubtedly hold beliefs that are both positive and empowering. Your beliefs will be an extension of your deepest self and ideally not represent any internal conflicts that you formed over the years.

For now it is worth appreciating that your thoughts, attitudes and beliefs work in harmony with one another. They are all contained within the same dimension and are forever supporting you toward successfully *Navigating Life.* Your beliefs affect and influence the other dimensions within the life wheel. Your predominant beliefs about money, health and well-being, relationships and your career are largely affected by your deeply held beliefs. This is because your beliefs are the filter from which you paint your reality. It is worth frequently examining your deepest beliefs to see if they are aligned and congruent with what you wish to manifest in your life.

Creating empowering beliefs should be an ongoing process that is aligned with the other seven dimensions. As you *Navigate Life* and your beliefs are disempowering you, you will begin to see evidence of this by moving from a *Navigating* state to a *Parked* state. It is important to understand that the nature of reality operates within the present moment and is relaying back your deeply held thoughts and beliefs. It makes sense that in order to change your external circumstances, turn inward and examine the unconscious thought process with the view of updating them.

As you begin to update and change your beliefs to more empowering ones, you will begin to see evidence of this as you move from a *Parked* state to *Navigating.* I suggest that you review and revise your beliefs on a monthly basis for reality has a chance to catch up with your thought process. This is a useful strategy since you remain ahead by not allowing your beliefs to lag, which are subsequently reflected in your external world.

When you are successfully *Navigating Life* all the components of your thoughts, beliefs and attitudes conspire and work together to create the ideal circumstances to manifest the life you dream of.

Emotions

Your emotions can serve to lift you to great heights or hinder your growth. One of the mechanisms which may become useful with managing your emotions is to become mindful of them as they occur. For many people, they remain asleep when it comes to the nature of their emotions and the role they serve in their life. By learning to identify and manage your emotions, you have a better understanding of how they best serve you. It takes time, patience and perseverance.

Examine your emotions. What emotions are serving you right now? Are they useful? In order to understand the emotion and possibly reframe it, you need to examine the belief behind it, for that is the fuel. If the emotion is one of sadness, anger or anxiety, look closely at whether it is serving your growth. The Buddhist principle states if the emotion is not necessary, drop it. Put it down as though it were a backpack. It is meant to be as simple as that, yet not quite so in practice.

If you find yourself flying off the handle when a loved one does the wrong thing by you, examine the emotion. Speak to it: *what do you want me to know or learn?* Look back to the belief surrounding the emotion. I can assure you that your loved one is not the cause or the trigger of your emotion. It is the meaning you attached to it when he/she forgot to ring you while they were traveling interstate on business. You attached a meaning and assigned an emotion to it, which served an outcome, whether positive or negative.

When you are in alignment with your inner self, you develop a deep understanding and relationship with self. Your emotions, thoughts and beliefs remain congruent with your inner wisdom. They serve you, rather than work against you. You develop inner peace, harmony, joy and bliss. You radiate passion, enthusiasm and those around you are drawn to you like a moth to a flame. Your emotional constitution has an impact on your overall state of well-being. You have no doubt been in a situation where emotions have got the better of you. It may have been a reactive situation based on anger or anxiety in which you reacted emotionally rather than taking the time to sit with the emotion.

People who *Navigate Life* have a greater understanding and awareness of their emotional constitution. This does not mean that they are not emotional beings. Instead, they learn to work with their emotional state rather than allowing the emotion to run wild. What is the point of runaway emotions hurtling out of control and not being able to master them when you need to? The person who successfully *Navigates Life* is aware of their predominant emotional state. They observe them as though they were standing on the edge of the shoreline watching the waves come in — some waves come crashing in, whilst others serenely meld into the shoreline.

The ocean waves are a good metaphor for your emotional state insofar as the tides are influenced by the earth's gravitational field and planetary alignments. Your emotional state is influenced by your predominant thoughts. The purpose of *Navigate Life* is to equip you with the awareness and resources to effectively mask your thoughts before they give rise to negative emotions.

For a moment reflect on a point in time when your emotions were out of control, much like a car skidding on ice. Recall the intensity of the emotion at the time and despite your best intentions to master the emotion, it was to no avail as the situation grew dire as time passed. A useful analogy may be the reference of trying to control the skidding car on ice by over braking and over steering. The more you overcompensate, the more the situation worsens.

It is for this reason that reasoning with people whilst they are in the throes of emotion is difficult. When pilots learn to fly, they rehearse a series of crash landings which are performed at the commencement of their tuition and toward the end of the class. The purpose of these drills is to automate the response in the likelihood that they must perform a crash landing. In such a situation, there is no time to think and it is best to delegate the role to the subconscious mind, which is devoid of analysis.

This is a useful example for understanding and managing your emotions insofar as when you come to terms with your worst emotional crisis, you are better equipped to take control and master the emotion before it takes you into a nosedive and hurtles out of control. By this time it is far too late to rectify the situation since an emotional intensity is absolute and cannot be reasoned with logical thought. This can be seen in everyday situations that relate to food or clothes. Depending on your likes you may have an emotional attraction toward certain foods, and despite your good intentions to avoid eating foods, such as cakes and biscuits, but your emotions reason differently when you are most vulnerable.

Navigate Life teaches you to understand and appreciate the highs and lows of your emotional being. When you observe your emotions like observing the waves crashing into the shoreline, you become less invested and attached to the emotions. You see that emotions will rise and fall and becoming attached to them is not conducive to your overall mental and emotional well-being.

Many people get stuck with a myriad of runaway emotions that they are unable to master. Whether they are in social situations, at work or at home with family, losing control can happen just about any time. Rather than getting stuck in this state, which we defined as being *Parked*, it is best to remain in a *Navigating* emotional state by being aware of the emotions to begin with.

By now you will note that the eight dimensions of the life wheel have been purposely constructed to perform a strong and sound wheel, when tensioned correctly, supports a solid structure.

All eight dimensions of the life wheel are an integrated whole, while operating individually they still work together in harmony by complementing one another. *Navigating Life* means *Navigating* successfully within each of those eight dimensions. I suggest you review the *Life Wheel* on a monthly basis by checking in to see which areas you may be *Parked* in. As indicated previously it is best to tend to a situation well before it makes its passage into your reality.

Motivational leaders talk about the concept of modeling behavior on those people who are successful. My suggestion to you is through regular examination you will begin to experience which of the eight dimensions you are successfully *Navigating* and model the behavior from that into your *Parked* dimensions. So for example, if your career is successful, yet as a result your health is in a *Parked* state then it is advisable that you model the behavior, the habits, the thoughts and practices from your career and channel it toward your health.

Chapter Summary

- There are eight dimensions within the *Navigate Life* framework.

- Like a well tensioned bicycle wheel, each area influences the other. It is imperative that you pay close attention to each of these eight houses as you *Navigate Life.*

- Your *Life View* is the strongest aspect of the eight dimensions and affects the other dimensions. It is representative of your overall level of consciousness.

- The purpose of the *Navigate Life wheel* is to be attuned to the areas that are lacking and undesirable. By repeatedly taking inventory of these eight dimensions, you are better equipped to effectively manage your life.

- What you value and give your attention to, will also increase in value with respect to that particular dimension.

- *Navigate Life* is a continual and perpetual journey. Where your attention and energy goes is represented or manifested in your external world.

- Your belief about reality shapes and colors your preview of future events. As within, so without.

- Many of your childhood programs are no longer useful nor valid as an adult, especially if left unexamined.

- In order to create a new future, it is important that you examine your childhood programs (beliefs) and create a new set of empowering beliefs that align with your anticipated future.

- Albert Einstein reminds us that, *you cannot solve a problem with the same level of thinking that created it.* We need to change our level of thought in order to create a new future.

- Life is not merely a cause and effect reality as many people are led to believe. You are the master of your destiny and have the power to influence your future more than you realise.

- By connecting with your inner most desires, you are well equipped to create a purposeful and meaningful life. This becomes an extension of your authentic self.

- Your relationship with others are a barometer of your self-worth.

- The majority of problems one faces in life can be attributed to three main areas: health, finance and relationships.

- You are repeatedly creating and maintaining relationships with others and yourself. It is said that you *coach* people on how to treat you.

- Life is a continual process of learning and growing. There is no need to get anywhere in a hurry. Do not be dissuaded when you make mistakes. Simply realign yourself with your intended outcome.

- Epigenetics has a greater influence on how our environment interacts and shapes our biology.

- Almost 70% of illness and disease can be prevented through better lifestyle choices.

- We are born with an abundance of energy and vitality. How we choose to use that will be determined by the lifestyle choices we make and the thoughts we repeatedly entertain.

- Your beliefs toward money is influenced by your values and beliefs. If you feel you are undeserving of money then it will be scarce in your life.

- Your internal dialogue around money creates either an abundance of it in your life or lack. Correct your inner dialogue and your outside world will follow.

- Being self-aware allows you to make conscious choices which are in alignment with your core needs and desires. They become an expression of your deeper self.

- Spirituality calls for the understanding that you are not just a human being comprised of flesh and bone. You are a multi-dimensional, spiritual being that is an expression of universal intelligence.

- *Self-awareness* and *spirituality* work synergistically with the other dimensions in an integrated manner to allow a unified and integrated union of the *Navigating Life* principles.

- Your *Attitude* is your gauge and barometer toward life. Your attitude is your driving force, and the engine that propels you forward in life

- We process approximately 60,000 – 70,000 thoughts a day. Many of these thoughts are on a feedback look, meaning we think the same stuff day in day out.

- Your thoughts influence your physiology. This is no more evident than when you receive bad news and your heart beat begins to dramatically rise.

- Your beliefs have the potential to shape your reality in a positive or negative way. Your beliefs are registered and stored within your subconscious mind.

- If left unexamined, your beliefs have the potential to cause you pain and suffering if they do not align with your intended future.

- Creating empowering beliefs should be an ongoing process that is aligned with the other seven dimensions.

- Your emotions have the power to color your life or cause misery and distress. It is how you respond to and interact with your emotions which determine success in life.

- Self-examination seeks to identify any wayward emotions which have been left unchecked. By regularly checking in, you are able to attend to any emotions which are not in keeping with how you wish to lead your life.

- When you are in alignment with your inner self, you develop a deep understanding and relationship with self. Therefore, your emotional constitution has an impact on your overall state of well-being.

- Tending to your emotions before they slide out of control like a hurtling car, may be a useful analogy for regularly attending to your inner state before it is too late.

CHAPTER EIGHT
Navigating Life Blueprint

Taking Inventory of Your Life:

Create Empowering Beliefs

> *"The outer conditions of a person's life will always be found to reflect their inner beliefs."*

James Allen

In the previous chapters we examined the nature of beliefs and the role beliefs play in successfully *Navigating Life*. In this chapter we will examine in greater detail how to reframe your beliefs. You will gain an understanding of how to examine your current set of beliefs with the purpose of creating **empowering beliefs**.

As stated previously, many of your beliefs were formed years ago and most of them during your formative years as a child. Beliefs are subsequently held within the subconscious mind where they are accepted as truth.

As we mature from our childhood to our adult years, the added maturity and life experiences begin to reshape our perceptions; we may begin to challenge formerly held beliefs. Many beliefs which are challenged and reexamined relate to religion, relationships, and universal truths. The limitation of our beliefs is attributed to the fact that they are always one-sided and based on a biased perception. It is for this reason beliefs should be updated as one's life experience changes.

How do you know if your current belief is an outdated belief or a limiting belief? The most obvious way is to look at your current circumstances and reality and if anything within that reality is not to your liking there is a limiting belief which has created those circumstances. For example, if you desire financial freedom, yet you are living in debt and from paycheck to paycheck, then your belief about money or financial responsibility may be outdated. It may be worthwhile to journal some of the beliefs that you created that relate to money.

We will examine this process in this chapter so you have a clear understanding on how to work through the process in order to create greater clarity. Allow me, however, to provide a caveat: Your beliefs may be lying dormant within your subconscious mind and in some instances may not been examined for years; there is a likelihood that examining them may accompany unwanted emotions. The emotion attached to the belief is a way of securing it to the subconscious mind.

If your belief came from someone close to you, like a parent or guardian, and you formed this belief at a young age, it is likely that you have attached it to an emotion in order for the belief to be more concrete, more real. When one examines the belief later in life, they are also examining the emotion which is attached to that belief. At a subconscious level, the emotion is linked to the belief, the belief is linked to the life of the guardian from which the belief came from. For this reason it is important that you move prudently as you undertake the self-examination process.

Examining and challenging beliefs is fundamental to successfully *Navigating Life* since it allows you to create the beliefs which are in alignment with your true self. Rather than the belief which is based on other's view, experience or perceptions. It is important that you form beliefs which are of *your* choosing. As you begin the process of examining your beliefs you may become aware of emotional centers within your body or experience the feeling of conflict. This is a healthy sign of progress and I urge you to continue working through the self-examination process, because you are on the verge of a breakthrough! The inner conflict is much like the process undertaken when you detoxify your body from certain foods. If you have ever eliminated coffee or alcohol from your diet, you no doubt felt the withdrawal effects of the substance leaving your body. Whilst it may be an undesirable effect, it is no doubt beneficial in order to purge yourself from toxic substances.

Unconscious Beliefs

Unconscious beliefs are powerful because this level of the mind operates as an automatic pilot function, accepting programming from the conscious mind. Your unconscious mind accepts the truth of any belief and does not question the belief since this is the domain of the conscious mind.

Whilst unconscious beliefs may initially prove daunting once brought to the conscious level, they are largely cloaked in misperception and can be unveiled for reexamination.

I have confronted *many* of the unconscious beliefs which were formed during my early childhood. For example, as a child I had a strong fear and dislike of water, which prevented me from taking swimming lessons with my classmates. I was so panic stricken at the thought of jumping into the deep end that my mother had to accompany me.

What appeared easy for most of my classmates, was as an insurmountable challenge for me to overcome. I still recall standing on the edge of the swimming pool, the swim instructor waiting in anticipation in the water, with arms outstretched ready to catch me as I jumped in.

The fear that overcame me at the time also shut down my physiological body functions. My heart beat escalated, my breathing became shallow and I still recall the tense tight feeling in my digestive system during the swim class and afterwards when I felt safe. It is no secret that as an adult I experienced bouts of irritable bowel syndrome which re-emerges when anxiety surfaces my life.

Fast forward many years later: As an adult I began working with a psychologist's office where I was also being mentored by this professional. During one of our sessions together I was regressed to my childhood to examine the basis of fear and where it began. It was no surprise that the fear was traced back to those swim classes.

I recall at the time of the swim classes that I had made a declaration in the belief. I declared that since I was unable to jump into the deep end like all the other children that I was no good and would never amount to anything. Now I know what you are thinking - what child of eight years old would know about forming such a belief? Yet ironically, I had declared to myself that I was no good and useless because I was comparing myself to the other children who were jumping—fearlessly—into the water.

This belief remained with me well into my adult life, appearing in the form of fear whenever a situation was out of my comfort zone. It was not until my mentoring sessions with the psychologist that I came face-to-face with my unconscious belief by deciding to examine it further with the view of overcoming it.

In essence, the childhood beliefs I had created when I compared myself to the other children had the potential to wreak havoc throughout my life if left unchecked.

The purpose of this chapter is to help you create empowering beliefs by becoming a conscious creator and *choosing* beliefs that are in harmony with your deepest self. It is for this reason that I repeat the mantra throughout this book: *know thyself.* The more you understand your core needs and your core beliefs, the better you are able to create the circumstances of your life that reflect your inner landscape.

In this next section we are going to examine a number of your beliefs. Re-writing the script of a belief is not as daunting as it may initially appear. What needs to be understood when creating a new belief system is that it must remain congruent with your deepest self. As you begin to examine and rewrite a new script for your beliefs, you will begin to notice emotions emerge, as was noted in earlier chapters.

Recall that an **emotion is simply energy in motion**. The emotion wishes to express itself through you and in doing so asks that you come along for the ride. As a passenger it is important that you do not interact with the emotion, for in doing so you give it energy. The greater the energy given to the emotion, the greater the impact it has upon your physiology. That is why I suggest that you learn to detach from the emotion by merely observing it and becoming aware of its nature.

Some useful questions to ask as you undertake this process are:

What does the emotion look or feel like?
Where do I feel the emotion within my body?
What does the emotion want me to do, be, act or become?

Let us now get to work by examining the emotions with the view of receiving information. Once again this process is one of self-discovery and self-realization. Under no circumstance do I suggest that you become intertwined with the emotion by labeling or judging the emotion. You are playing the role of a detective or sleuth by uncovering what unconscious or repressed beliefs reside deep within the subconscious mind and in order to become aware of them.

A word on observing emotions and thoughts: many people have a hard time understanding the concept of the *observer*. Observing thoughts or an emotion simply denotes remaining detached from the experience and observing it as you would waves coming in to the shore line. As noted in the earlier chapters, I used the example of waves by drawing the analogy to your thoughts and emotions. If you continue with that analogy in this exercise it will become useful in order for you to gain a deeper understanding and awareness of what is being revealed.

The simple way to become an efficient observer is the following example. Close your eyes for a moment and imagine there is a beautiful meal that has been placed in front of you. The setting is perfect since you are in your favorite restaurant and the hustle and bustle of the restaurant entices you to feel at peace. You are dining with a loved one and the mood and the ambiance allows you to savor every moment.

The lights are dim and the conversation between you and your loved one is pleasant and engaging. You could not wish to be anywhere else at this point in time. Now, hopefully your eyes were closed during this exercise and you got a feel for what it was like to be in this setting.

While you were imagining this experience with your eyes closed, were you aware of any mental conversations taking place in your mind? Hopefully, you observed the experience and savored every moment by embodying the emotions that were recalled. This is what we mean when we talk about *becoming the observer*. We are easily able to observe experiences via the use of our imagination with our eyes closed. There is no reason why you cannot adapt the same skills toward observing your thoughts and emotions.

As you undertake this upcoming exercise, if you become unsettled or feel uneasy with the observation process, I suggest you return to the exercise above. Do not push or antagonize yourself at any point during this process, however, you may need to overcome discomfort in revealing answers which will allow you the opportunity to begin your deeper work.

Okay. Let's begin delving into our work. Firstly, it is of value categorizing your beliefs according to the following list:

- Money and finances
- Relationships
- Career and business
- Universal truths
- Personal
- Other

In order to get the best out of your self-examination process, it is best that you undertake this at a quiet time when you are not rushed. Personally, I have noted the best times of the day are generally the morning and the evenings, since the subconscious mind is most impressionable at these times.

Label a heading with one of the six categories listed above. In this manner you are able to define the nature of the belief by associating it to a category. This will allow you to create new and empowering beliefs in place of your outdated beliefs.

Under the heading of money and finances, write down any limiting or disempowering beliefs that you hold toward money. How will you know that your beliefs are limiting? Limiting beliefs normally consist of direct statements in the negative sense. When examined in the right setting, they can illicit an emotional charge within your body.

To test this, try this simple exercise for a moment. Declare a statement that you know to be true and note the intensity of the emotion that emanates from your body. Your statement might be something along the lines of, "I love my husband John. He is my soul mate and the father of my three beautiful children."

As you made that declaration you no doubt would have experienced a light and tingling feeling somewhere in your body. Where was that feeling situated? Was it in the front of your body, in your chest or stomach? Note how it felt? Was it light and empowering?

Concurrently, if you were to make a disempowering statement you would also have an emotion and feeling to that statement. Your body is much like a finely tuned receiving and sending signal. It is continually alerting you to the validity of your statements through the power of feelings. These feelings reside within specific centers (chakras) of your body that are designed to alert you to the consistency and alignment of your thoughts with your deepest self.

Begin with this heading at the top of your page: *Money* and *Finances.* Write down any beliefs that you may have heard during your lifetime, or beliefs that you personally consider to be true relating to money and finances.

To help you with this process I have included some statements below which relate to money and finances that you may have heard when growing up. These are general in nature and should only be used as a template or guide to help you recall your own beliefs. Do not be concerned with getting it right at this stage, since there is no right or wrong in this process. This exercise is about extracting and dumping information from your subconscious mind onto the page. What you think may be an incorrect belief may look different on paper. Persist with this process, even if doubts and insecurities arise.

Money doesn't grow on trees!

I do not have enough money to meet my financial commitments.

Money is the root of all evil.

Rich people are greedy and dishonest.

The more money I have, the more problems are likely to accompany them.

If I have a lot of money, I will alienate many of my friends and family who may become jealous.

I am not worthy of receiving all this money.

Making and accumulating money is not spiritual.

As you can see from the statements above, they are limiting statements about money. They are limiting since there is no basis or validity to the belief. I could easily find a handful of spiritual people who are wealthy, yet donate much of their wealth toward charities and greater causes to disprove such beliefs.

You may have noted at this point that your beliefs are purely based on your perception. Your perception is based on your experiences. To orchestrate this example in a different way, we could easily take another person and put them in your position and ask them to hold the same beliefs. A belief can be challenged by finding a person who believes the opposite.

The purpose and nature of beliefs when they are aligned with your deepest self has the potential to ignite your deepest realizations. Your beliefs are a preview of the coming attractions that you wish to manifest in your life. Dr Wayne Dyer wrote a book appropriately named, *You'll See it When You believe It*. The book reveals that what you hold deep within your unconscious mind has the power to manifest in your life.

In modern day society we have been conditioned to see something first and then believe it. This probably stems from a scientific-based mindset which relies on the proof of physical reality. I would argue that there are many things that we cannot see which we still accepted as realities in life. Love is a foremost example, because it is neither tangible nor can it be scientifically examined or explained. Yet, hopefully, we have all experienced love at some point in our lives and know and accept it as a real experience. .

In life, there are many things that are unaccounted for scientifically, but nonetheless they exist. Though maybe not explained or scientifically proven—your beliefs exist—yet if you hold disempowering beliefs, the net effect is that your life circumstances will be a reflection of whatever you believe at the deepest level.

After you have written your beliefs down, take time to reflect upon them as this permits the subconscious mind to work on your statements. This happens through images, words or feelings. Be attentive in the coming days for anything that might emerge that sparks your attention. You might have a dream that evening that relates to your belief. If so, your subconscious mind is advising you on the best possible resolution to create a new empowering belief or it may provide you with more resources to help you better understand the belief.

When working with the mind, nothing is linear—the mind does not work in logic. It works in abstract and fragmented puzzles. When understood correctly, it has the power to reveal to you the information you need to heal your life situation—so be attentive!

The next phase is to create the new empowering belief. For a new belief to be accepted by the subconscious mind, it needs to be believable. There is no point creating a belief that does not resonate with your deepest self. While you consciously and logically might believe it to be true, your subconscious mind might have another view of it. The subconscious mind is experienced at its job since it has been doing it for many years and is accustomed to listening out for beliefs which do not make sense.

Most practitioners or coaches suggest the use of Muscle Testing, otherwise known as kinesiology, to test the belief. While it has many merits, I believe there are still too many variances that affect the outcome, especially if the person is untrained. For this reason, I suggest you avoid this practice despite what literature suggest, as it remains far too an inaccurate measure for the novice.

The method I prefer is journaling. It is based in the classical approach for analysis and can be very effective for helping create new beliefs. Journaling requires that you connect with your inner self through silent witnessing and observation to create the new belief. After you have written down a limiting belief and taken time to ponder it, return to your journal, and under the limiting belief, write down the new belief. Do not rush this process. I suggest that you find some quiet time in which to do this exercise. The quiet time allows you to silently listen, feel and intuitively gauge the response that is brought forward.

Under the limiting belief, write a new belief that challenges it. Remember, it must sound convincing and believable otherwise it will not be accepted, despite your intentions to think it sounds valid.

Let us work through the first three money beliefs on the previous pages, by creating new empowering beliefs alongside them. Obviously your beliefs will differ to the ones given in the book. These are only a guide.

Limiting Belief:
Money doesn't grow on trees.

Empowering Belief:
I attract all the money I need with ease and perfection. I create an abundance mentality when I think about money.

Limiting Belief:
I do not have enough money to meet my financial commitments.

Empowering Belief:
I always have more than enough money to meet my financial obligations. When I align with my deepest self, the financial resources I need easily show up in my life.

Limiting Belief:
Money is the root of all evil.

Empowering Belief:
Money is an energy source, which is attracted to me easily and effortlessly. I am now in alignment with the energy of money.

As you can see from the new empowering beliefs on the previous page, there is a lighter feeling to the statement, which is not clothed in negativity or biased perception. In many cases, when creating new beliefs you will initially find them to be neutral with an unbiased perspective. This is appealing to the subconscious mind since there are no overlapping beliefs which contradict or challenge the new belief.

It will take some time for you to get used to creating new beliefs. At first, it may seem like *mumbo jumbo* and unclear, but as you persist you will find that they just seem to flow onto the paper from your pen. This is the optimal way to create the beliefs since they become an extension of the mind.

I suggest you repeat the self-examination process when you observe changes in your external circumstances. Beliefs consist of layers, which are clustered together, meaning they are linked or tied together in similar groupings. Since beliefs are clustered together, when you have changed one belief, other similarly held beliefs are also modified or abandoned.

Be patient with the self-examination process. I suggest you do not expect too much from this process, but use it as an opportunity to become better acquainted with yourself. By learning and discovering new aspects of your inner landscape, you become better equipped to create new and empowering beliefs for the future, rather than repeat toxic and negative cycles. How will you know that your thoughts are out of alignment? Look to your outside world as your barometer of whether you are *Navigating Life* or *Parked*.

Chapter Summary:

- Many of your current beliefs were created during your formative years, in childhood, and were influenced by loved ones and those in positions of authority.

- Beliefs are held within the subconscious mind where they are accepted as truth.

- Your current view of reality is testament to whether the nature of your beliefs is bringing you what you desire.

- It is important to examine your beliefs if you feel they do not serve you. Self-examination is one method of testing the validity of the beliefs.

- Unconscious beliefs may surface later in life to allow you to come face-to-face with the belief, as a means of examining the deepest part of you.

- You have the power to create empowering beliefs by changing the inner dialogue and script pertaining to the belief.

- Assigning a positive emotion to the belief saturates it with an emotional intensity that is appealing to the subconscious mind.

- Learn to witness or observe your emotions by detaching from creating a story around it. Become the silent witness. Recognize that outdated beliefs are merely a call to examine an aspect of yourself that you created long ago. Review and revise the belief regularly to see if it aligns with your current view of reality.

- Create new empowering beliefs via the use of muscle testing with a trained practitioner. Otherwise use it as a guide only. Follow through with journaling instead.

CHAPTER NINE

Navigating Life Blueprint

Navigate Your Emotional Wellbeing

Master Your Emotions

The Nature of Emotions

> *"When we direct our thoughts properly, we can control our emotions."*
> W. Clement Stone

In the previous chapter we looked at aspects of negative belief patterns and their potential to create undesired circumstances in your life. We touched briefly on the nature of emotions and how your emotions are inextricably linked to your thoughts and beliefs.

As noted in earlier chapters, emotions are energy in motion. An emotion is the expression of your innermost thoughts. Your emotions serve as a guide and instrument in order to help you successfully *Navigate Life*. Without emotions you would not have a gauge of whether your thoughts are aligned with truth. When you experience an emotion, it is expressed through a part or parts of your body, which provide you with either a positive feeling or a negative feeling. Either way, you are simply *Navigating Life* or remaining *Parked*.

Your emotions serve as a means of self-correcting your thought process in order to live in alignment with your deepest self. Your emotions help you to become better acquainted with what you truly desire to experience.

They are not meant to create states of anguish, nor are they meant to cripple you. When you understand the mechanism of how an emotion advises you that you are either aligned with your deepest self or moving away from the deepest self, you will gain a greater understanding in order to self-regulate your thought process.

Your emotions are an energy system that moves through the body. This is an important distinction to understand since emotions may become lodged within certain points of your body and cause a host of negative physiological functions. The two emotions of anxiety and anger have been linked to back pain. Dr. John Sarno, a prominent medical doctor, wrote a book in the early seventies called Healing Back Pain. Dr. Sarno coined the term Tension Myoneural Syndrome or TMS. TMS is defined as mild oxygen deprivation of spinal nerves or tendons. The pain is generally psychosomatic and may be initiated by the pressures of life and particular personality characteristics.

Dr. Sarno details in his work, that when he began to work with emotion's of his patients, the pain which they experienced as either back pain or other related body aches and pains, normally disappear in the ensuing weeks or months. He hypothesized that since emotions are an expression of energy, it is common for the emotion to become lodged within a body system as a means of alerting the person to deal with the emotion.

His work highlights the importance of understanding our emotions in order to *Navigate Life*. That said, there seems to be a gender division on what it means as to how one's emotions are handled. Traditionally speaking, women are generally better equipped to deal with their emotional constitution before it escalates into something bigger; this is one example of their emotional intelligence. Women have a better emotional guidance system and have learned from childhood how to effectively manage their emotions. Despite the accusation from the opposite sex that women are *too* emotional, their range of emotionality merely illustrates the complexity of the female brain in this region.

Conversely, most men have not grown up with this same awareness of their emotional states and tend to repress or shove the emotions deep down, believing that in doing so they might go away. Men's left brain thinking orientates them toward logic more than the right brain, intuitive and emotional states. It is for this reason that men and women in intimate relationships may find it challenging to relate to one another since women process from an emotional, or feeling context, while men process from the area of the brain that focuses on rational thinking.

As a result, men are more likely to experience psychosomatic illnesses since they are more prone to repressing or neglecting their emotions. Emotions want to be heard; they will do whatever it takes to draw your awareness. Neglecting your emotions, believing that they will go away, is like pushing against a sumo wrestler in the hope of pushing him out of the ring. Undoubtedly, the more you neglect the emotion, the more the emotion will push back on you until your awareness is drawn to the emotion until you take action and make it conscious.

Emotions serve as a means of drawing your attention to an aspect of yourself that requires examination. For example, if you were bullied and harassed as a child and teenager, you may experience negative emotions of low self-worth and self-doubt. These emotions serve to remind you of your self-worth. Your emotions serve as valuable tools that provide you with information in relation to your ability to *Navigate Life*. When you are in harmony and aligned with your emotions you are *Navigating Life* successfully. Those who remain *Parked* are blind to their emotions, believing that they will simply go away if ignored.

Your emotions cannot be ignored. As illustrated via the sumo wrestler analogy, you can see that the more you resist the emotion, the more the emotion attempts to move its way through you. Many people are struck down by the intensity of the neglected or repressed emotions which may surface at an inopportune time. There are many cases of busy corporate executives who have been struck down with unexplained psychosomatic illnesses, attributed to aspects of the mind.

Western medicine is only now beginning to understand the mind-body interconnectedness. A branch of medicine known as psychoneuroimmunology deals with the brain and nervous system and immune system function. As the levels of stress continue to rise in our lives, the relationship this has on the mind and body may be reflected in the number of unexplained illnesses being presented to doctors across the globe. Chronic fatigue and adrenal fatigue are now considered to be first world illnesses that are largely attributed to the ever-increasing stresses imposed on modern man.

What does all this have to do with understanding and managing your emotions? If left unchecked, your emotions become an accomplice to the stress response and in no time your body has learnt to initiate stress chemicals every time you entertain stressful thoughts. The key element to understand in this section is that your emotions are more complex than you believe. It is essential that you become better acquainted with your emotions by tuning in to how you feel.

An effective approach to checking-in may be as simple as asking yourself, *how am I doing?* A simple statement like this renders an impulse to the unconscious mind awakening any dormant thoughts or emotions that need to be examined. The more you practice posing questions to your mind, the better you become at developing a two-way relationship. You become a better listener and observer of the emotions since you become aware of the language in which the emotion renders itself.

The Observer

You might recall in the previous chapter I asked you to observe or witness your thoughts as they relate to limiting beliefs. We discussed the idea that you undertake this process when you close your eyes and use your imagination. We used the example of being in a restaurant and have a plate of food before you and observe the scenery unfolding in front of you.

Observing your emotions is much the same as observing your thoughts, yet you use a different sensory awareness which requires training. When observing a thought, you are listening to words being played out in your mind in the sound of your own voice. As stated earlier, this is a language that you become efficient in the more you practice it.

Observing an emotion is a little more complex than listening to your thoughts. Since emotions are feeling based, you will now be required to understand and become aware of how your emotions feel. Let us take a detailed look into how you improve tuning in to your emotions. Remember that becoming the observer of the emotions benefits you insofar as you are using consciousness in order to draw awareness to the emotion.

Awareness is continually present in your life, it is just that we add a narrative to the awareness in order to understand what we are seeing. An example of this might be taking your dog for a walk in the park and observing the other dog owners. Your consciousness observes the different breeds of dogs as well as the owners. It tunes into the sound of dogs when they bark and the way they interact with their owners. However, if your mind intervenes by adding a narrative to the observation, recalling information that you have previously observed at some point in your life.

Your mind is a database of events and experiences that it calls upon in order to predict what it sees in the present moment or what it anticipates might unfold in a future occurrence. By observing your emotions you are unlearning and silencing much of that internal dialogue that has served you for much of your life. I am not suggesting that the process is easy, nor that you will be able to turn off the incessant internal chatter, but rather that you will become better acquainted with your ability to observe via consciousness.

Once you have asked *yourself how am I doing?* you will be guided toward either a series of thoughts or feelings. Do not label or judge whatever surfaces, instead, notice whether it is a strong impulse framed as either a thought or an emotion. If it is a thought, use the technique explained in the previous chapter by observing the dialogue. Do not become invested in the thought by creating a conversation around it. Doing so will give more energy to it and that is what we wish to avoid.

Observing emotions is a slightly different process in that it is feelings orientated. Many people have a difficult time being aware of the somatic responses that their bodies given them. Learning to become aware of physical sensations and responses within your human form is a matter of practice and takes time and discipline. Do not let this dissuade you from continuing the process. Nothing good can be gained in a short amount of time.

Let us use an example to illustrate how to draw awareness to emotional centers within the body. Suppose you are driving to work one day and having had a rough start to the day you are running late. In your frantic state you decide to drive a little faster than what the speed limit mandates. While this was a momentary lapse of judgment, you soon hear the siren of a police vehicle asking you to pull over. You are torn between the frustration, anxiety, and anger. Your heart begins to beat rapidly and in your mind; you begin to form a number of plausible explanations that hopefully will get you out of this traffic offence. It is to no avail and the police officer issues you with a $300 speeding offence. You begrudgingly take the ticket and as you drive off, you start thinking about all the bills that you have to pay that month and how you really did not need to get this speeding ticket.

Despite all this you managed to get to work on time and after your morning coffee, you are now feeling a little better about the incident. The beauty of hindsight is that we are able to rationally look at the emotional situation that earlier caused you to feel a flutter of raging thoughts and emotions. In your calm and relaxed state you are now better equipped to rationalize the thought process, instead of reacting.

In order to become emotionally intelligent, you must learn to train that aspect which initiates the flooding of thoughts and emotions before they happen. The next time you are angry is possibly not the best time to practice being aware of your thoughts and emotions.

Returning to the earlier example of the speeding ticket – since you experienced a number of thoughts and emotions at the time, it can be well-meaning in terms of how you respond to the situation. It is worth repeating that it is not in your best interest to create a dialogue with the thought process going on in your mind. Your best response each time is to just stand back in your mind and observe the thoughts and emotional process. Do not become invested in the drama unfolding within you.

There is an axiom in neuropsychology which states that *neurons that fire together wire together*. What this effectively means is that when you give more thought energy to a situation, you create more packets of information in the brain which creates more neurons firing together, thus building a greater network for the thought process to unfold. Witnessing the thoughts or the emotion disengages you from becoming embroiled in this situation and does not initiate neural connections.

In receiving the speeding ticket you may have noticed a combination of emotions ranging from anxiety, frustration and anger. It is best to practice these emotional responses in a calm setting, when you are in a parasympathetic state. This denotes the rest and digestive branch of your autonomic nervous system.

So let us look at the three main emotions which you felt during that interaction with the police officer:

Anxiety

Where in your body did you feel the anxiety? Or another way may be expressed by asking wherein your body were you *aware* of the anxiety? By phrasing the question in this manner you detach yourself from the emotion because you are not identifying yourself as the participant of the emotion. Rather you are framing it in your mind as someone having the experience of an anxious emotion somewhere in the body.

As you journal, you write down key elements that you recalled from the incident that occurred earlier. You are not playing the role of a psychoanalyst at this stage, but rather observing key emotional points from the incident. You are the emotional detective merely taking notes.

Some things you wish to record may include the location of the anxiety. Was the feeling situated in your stomach, in your chest, in your throat or anywhere else in your body? These main areas within the human form are considered to be focal chakra landmarks which absorb and hold onto emotional energy.

Let us say you felt anxiety within your stomach. *What did the anxiety feel like?* If you had to describe it in terms of painting a picture, what shape would the anxiety take? People often report anxiety as being a constricting feeling. When prompted they described anxiety as being like a vice slowly constricting them and subsequently causing a plethora of unwanted emotions. The better you become at attaching images to your feelings, the better you are able to navigate your way through these emotions the next time they emerge.

Once you have given an image to the anxiety and you have noted its location within your body, it is time to disengage from the process by breathing your way into the emotion. This process allows you to become centered and in the present moment, rather than allowing the runaway emotion to take hold of you.

The process of observation allows you to be present and grounded within the present moment by noticing and observing the emotion and its intensity within your body. The beauty of this process is that you become better equipped to notice and observe any untoward emotion which presents itself in the future. Self-examination through observation is a process of detachment since you are not attempting to do anything with the emotion but observe it and become aware of it.

Typically, anxiety has a particular feeling or energy about it since it is a combination of nervous tension and stress energy. People often feel anxious in situations which are beyond their control. This might include the fear of heights or crowded public places. Consciously, the person is mindful of the anxiety that is building up within, yet they are unable to trip the mind into releasing the anxiety. The purpose of observation allows you to notice without assigning meaning to the emotion and subsequently by breathing into the area of the body, the emotion is able to transmute.

Frustration

Frustration is also an emotion which accompanies anxiety and anger as it is a blend of the two emotions. When people feel frustrated, there is a sense of anger about not being able to find a solution to the situation and subsequently anxiety attaches itself to frustration due to the sense of not being in control.

The key is to be aware of the energy of frustration and what it looks like to you. The more you practice these exercises, the better you become at identifying and understanding the nature of the emotions, so that when and if they resurface, you will be in a position of power to work with them rather than have to take you by surprise.

Reverting back to the previous example of receiving the infringement ticket by the police officer, you may have noticed the frustration which emerged within your body. Often times you may experience more than one emotion at the same time and therefore it becomes difficult to know which emotion you are dealing with at the time.

My suggestion is that you not concern yourself with labeling or identifying whether you are angry, frustrated or anxious, rather you become acquainted with how the emotion feels and what it looks like in your mind. Undertaking this process creates a template and image sequence in your mind that is able to identify with the emotion when it emerges in the future.

Going through the same process as anxiety, identify what the emotion looks like to you as an image. Give it a color and a shape. What does it most resemble that is familiar to you? If you had a paintbrush with colors, what image would you paint the frustration? Is it a dark ominous color that looks like a cloud or is it a sense of tug-of-war type image of two opposing forces?

There is no right or wrong in your observation of frustration, although it is important that you become acquainted with the intensity of frustration and which body area it is located. You will notice in time that frustration tends to occupy the same area within your body. If you noticed frustration in your chest, it is likely that that is where you hold frustration.

As we used earlier with anxiety, observe the intensity of the emotion and note whether it is increasing, remaining neutral or de-creasing in intensity. As you perform your breathing exercises, use your awareness to breathe into the area of the body where the frustration is situated. Do not try to remove the frustration by breathing into it, since it is less likely that you will achieve success with this method.

As you continue to breathe into the frustration, become aware of whether the intensity of the emotion diminishes. What is happening to your thought process at the same time while you are aware of the emotion? At times your thoughts will be hurtling out of control, while the emotion runs away from you, and you may subsequently be dealing with two different components which may overwhelm you.

Frustration can be a positive emotion if you learn to work with it by understanding the nature of the emotion and reframing it. Frustration emerges within us in order to teach us that our thinking is out of alignment with our wants, desires, and needs. When you are happy and content, you are less frustrated than when you are pursuing a goal or a mission. The frustrated mind is attempting to rectify or change a situation believing that in doing so it will bring joy, happiness or peace to the individual. This is possibly the biggest misconception and the root cause of many people's suffering. The truth is that whatever experience you have in *any* given moment, it has been orchestrated perfectly by universal intelligence in order that you grow as a person.

With the help of these exercises and through repetition, you will find that the things, events or circumstances that once frustrated you, now have a little or no impact. This reveals a development within your consciousness as your mind expands to higher thresholds of thought. Therefore, frustration may be a teacher and an internal landmark that guides you toward becoming a stronger individual, capable of dealing with a variety of emotions.

It is almost certain that you will experience all these three emotions repeatedly throughout your life. The better you become equipped and understand them, the more peaceful, joyous and fulfilling your life will become.

Anger

Anger is one of the hardest emotions to tame since it may be considered one of the most aggressive emotions due to its intensity. When you feel anger, it is absolute and there is no denying the emotion. Attempting to talk your way out of it is usually to no avail since the emotion has a score to settle.

When you are caught up in the midst of anger, it is as though every other body system shuts down in order that the anger is heard. The ferocity in which it envelops the body is mirrored by the way people usually feel helpless to overcome it in the midst of the rage. Anger releases a myriad of toxic chemicals into the body which can inhibit and shut down body organs. The stress response to the human body is measured over time as the individual is repeatedly subjected to the fight or flight response. Nature never intended that we activate the response mechanism continually in our lives, yet for some people, this becomes a learned response and they find themselves stuck in a feedback loop.

Trying to attend to anger when you are in the throes of a full-blown rage is futile, so it is important that you practice and deal with anger when you are in relaxed state, Commonly referred to as "rest or digest response," or the parasympathetic branch of the Autonomic Nervous System, ANS. Only one branch of the ANS system can be activated at a time. This would be like attempting to sleep while simultaneously running away from danger. The ANS can only allocate energy toward one branch at a time.

Here is a helpful technique, similar to the frustration and anxiety techniques, which can be practiced at home and in a quiet and peaceful setting. The more you practice this technique, the more aware you will become of the nature of anger when it emerges. These exercises help draw your awareness to the language of toxic emotions. While I am not encouraging toxic emotions, we are engaging our emotions to become better equipped to deal with them when they emerge. Sometimes this can come out of nowhere and once the storm has settled and we have hurt loved ones, it is usually a little too late for apologies or remorse.

While sitting in a comfortable position, become aware of an angry moment you recently experienced. Close your eyes and run through the scene in your mind while being present in your body. Feel the emotion by amplifying it, that is, allow the energy of the emotion to be turned up so loud that it feels as though it will engulf you.

During this exercise it is important that you observe the feelings that arise without assigning meaning to them. We are not playing the detective or sleuth at this stage, but merely making notes on what we feel within the body.

> *Where in your body do you feel the anger?*
>
> *What does the anger look and feel like? Give it a name, a feeling and intensity?*
>
> *What is it asking of you? If you were talking to it and having a conversation, what would the emotion be saying?*

During this exercise, the emotion of anger may feel overwhelming and your response may be to withdraw from it. You may relive any negative feelings or emotions that were experienced during the time of the interaction. Return to the emotion of anger and avoid getting drawn into a discussion which occurred during the interaction.

As you answer the questions above, you may begin to notice the intensity present in your anger. If you have been suppressing this anger for many years, it is likely that the anger may be large and looking to express itself through your body. The purpose of this exercise is not to psychoanalyses the anger, but through mindfulness and compassion, allow yourself to uncover what the emotion is seeking to communicate to you.

When emotions are suppressed they build in intensity over time which can impact other body systems. This can cause psychosomatic illnesses which arise as a result of suppressing the emotion or neglecting to face it head on. The truth of the matter is that many people have suppressed, consciously or unconsciously, childhood emotions. Through counseling, individuals often report certain moments during their childhood when a loved one or parent/guardian denied them an experience, thus causing an angry moment.

While we often deflect such moments, believing that we do not need to face the emotion, our bodies have other intentions. Our bodies know the truth of our experiences and responds accordingly. There is no denying it. For this reason when you truly like something, you experience that emotion deep within the cells of your body. As researcher Candice Pert states in her book, Molecules of Emotion, "your body is your subconscious mind." (Pert, 1999) It knows the truth of your being and the nature of what you experience. Denying this is to deny the truth of your experience. The body does not lie and interacts and communicates with the mind to create experiences that reflect your perception and experience.

Your human form is your antenna for the way in which you experience your reality. There is no denying the truth of what it experiences and what it calls the truth. The key is to be aware by noticing and observing sensations in your body and matching them with mental and emotional constructs. When there are moments which stand out, investigate them through compassion and understanding. That is, be kind to yourself by silently witnessing the nature of the emotion and the messages that surface.

Naturally, your body will alert you to an incident which you have forgotten, repressed, or denied. It is seeking expression of that emotion in order to allow you to experience it. There is always a message contained within the nature of the emotion.

Chapter Summary:

- Our emotions reflect your predominant thoughts. Watch and observe your thoughts in order to become attuned to the ebb and flow of your emotional state.
- Emotions are capable of causing physiological disturbances

within the human body if left unchecked. Allow emotions to express themselves by becoming a silent witness; observe through compassion and love.

- Our emotions are a call to heal an aspect of yourself which you have repressed or denied.

- Use the *Checking-In* model of asking a simple question to oneself: *How am I doing?* Notice what arises—feelings or thoughts—and be present with them. Do not try to change them.

- Use the *Observer* method by noticing and being aware of where in your body is the emotion situated. *What does it feel like? What is it asking of you?*

- Use the example of anxiety, frustration and anger as a guide to identify and witness the emotions within the body. *Is it in the chest, throat, head or stomach? What does the energy feel or look like?*

- Examine: *Could there be hidden meaning behind the emotion you are experiencing? What would life look like without that emotion? Who would you be? Could it be a call to action?*

CHAPTER TEN

Navigate Your Emotional Well-being

Connect With Your Heart and Mind

> *"The greatest need of our time is to clean out the enormous mass of mental and emotional rubbish that clutters our minds."*

Thomas Merton

There is no denying the fact that life has become increasingly challenging. Living in a modern world is fraught with all manner of obstacles and hurdles, which restricts a person from being his/her authentic self. The stress of our modern existence means that we are dealing with an assortment of modern-day obstacles, many of which did not exist 100 years ago. The mental and emotional costs to a person can be represented by the amount of over-the-counter medication that is being prescribed. Everyone is searching for a quick fix. It seems that this ideology has been impressed upon us in our modern day life. Yet as human beings attending to our lives in this manner, it does not seem to offer the same reward as we might think.

We have said that we process anywhere between 60,000 to 70,000 thoughts a day. Many of these thoughts are on a feedback loop and are recurring thoughts. I also suggested that you try to recall your last original thought.

The incessant chatter and the monkey mind which prevails between our ears is the main cause of suffering these days. The reason being is that many people buy into the notion that because the thoughts are taking place in their mind, they must be real and therefore engage with the thought rather than observe it. We also looked at the observer effect which states that **you are not your thoughts, rather you are the witness of the thought process occurring within your mind.**

So if many people accept and engage with their thought process, what happens to the sound of the heart? Now you might be thinking that the heart does not have a voice, nor have you learnt the language of the heart in order to commune with it. You might be interested to know that the heart has a frequency which is fifty thousand times greater than your brain's frequency. Research has shown that the heart responds to the outside world well before the brain has time to respond.

What this means, is that we are only using one aspect of the human physiology to interact with our external world. Many people process their external life with their mind by attempting to draw meaning or attach a story, which in many instances is based on past conditioning and perception.

The heart does not have the same bias as the mind and therefore operates independently, whilst also working concurrently with the brain by sending its subtle messages. Your heart speaks in quiet whispers. It is for this reason that many people find it challenging to learn the language of the heart, because they have been conditioned to listen to the internal dialogue of the mind. Further to this, given our lives' have become hectic and chaotic, there is more noise in our external world which means retreating in silence has become increasingly difficult.

You may have come across programs and other self-help books that espouse the benefits and virtue of meditation to silence the mind. Many of my clients and audience members struggled transitioning into pure silence via meditation. Often it can take up to six months to one year to condition the mind to be in silence for thirty minutes or more. If you contemplate that your mind is active for at least twelve hours or more on any given day, it makes sense that learning to quiet the mind takes time and patience. Whilst I agree that meditation brings with it many lasting benefits, both mental, emotional and physiological, it is still impractical for busy people to find thirty minutes or more each day to sit in silence.

Mindfulness and meditation gurus suggest that thirty minutes is the minimum time required to bring the mind into silence. A good practice may be twice a day, once in the morning and last thing in the evening in order to gain greater understanding and awareness of the benefits of meditation.

Many people give up on meditation well into the first few weeks of the practice. It seems that sitting in silence, alone for anything more than ten minutes is enough to drive them crazy. This is largely attributed to the incessant, monkey mind which is being played out within the brain. Sitting alone in silence means listening to these thoughts repeatedly. But it does not have to be that way. Learning to meditate may also invite an opportunity to do so throughout your day without necessarily devoting one hour to being in pure silence.

Silence for many people seems to be a difficult undertaking for a multitude of reasons but primarily because there is much external noise taking place in our lives. It is because of this that one should find time to eliminate external silence regularly throughout the week. Being alone in silence allows the mind and body to harmonize with one another. It decelerates the stress response taking place in our body and moves us from a sympathetic state to a parasympathetic state.

As you recall in earlier chapters, we spoke about the balance or the yin and yang elements complementing one another. Your body cannot thrive in a stressed state since in doing so it gets locked into a sympathetic state – otherwise known as the fight or flight response. The physiological effects on your mind and body may be felt for prolonged periods of this repeated stress cycle. It is important that you seek time out of your busy life and reconnect with your inner self.

One of the ways in which you can approach this is to retreat into silence for as little as ten minutes at a time, spread throughout the day. I would advise that you get outside in nature if the temperature and weather is suitable. If you work in a busy corporate environment, a simple ten minute break to go outside and walk around the block can do wonders for your mind and body. If this is not an option, perhaps retreating to a quiet room and sitting alone in silence without the distraction of technological devices would do well to allow you to feel at peace with yourself.

I am well aware that our lives have become increasingly chaotic. Whether you are a stay-at-home mother or working in a stressful corporate environment, there appears to be very little time throughout one's day to be alone in silence. Many of you are probably undertaking some form of health fitness regime that might include cardiovascular exercise, resistance training or some form of yoga or Pilates. The point is that you have learned to condition and train your physical body by undertaking this form of exercise.

Conditioning and taming your mind is no different than training your physical body. In many cases it requires consistent persistence and discipline in order to reap the benefits. One of the easily recognized benefits of going into regular silence is an inner peace and harmony which opposes the chaos of your external world. This means that even though the chaos continues, such as emails, phone calls, deadlines and family pressures, you will find that these external occurrences have less impact on your inner world. What previously set you off and caused frustration and anxiety, will now have little impact on you.

If you struggle to find ten minutes of silence throughout your day, you might even use your commute home or to work as an opportunity to be in silence. Far too many people use electronic music devices to drown out the silence during their commute. Observe the number of people with a device plugged into their ears listening to loud music to drown out what is essentially silence.

I suggest you to take this time to put away your music device and just be with yourself. Run through the exercises listed in the previous chapters by asking yourself a simple question of *how am I doing?* or an even better one *how am I feeling?* Use this time to reconnect with yourself, through your inner world and become aware of the inner landscape and what it is asking of you. Doing so on a consistent basis means that you become aware of your emotional constitution and that you also notice and attend to any untoward thoughts or toxic emotions which may begin to surface.

As you become more comfortable sitting in silence, you will develop a language with your heart. Given that our minds are forever processing repeated thoughts from the previous day, it makes sense to go down there and connect with your heart to feel the energy stirring within. At first you might find this process daunting, since many people report that they are unable to hear anything.

When communing with your heart you will develop a unique language which is unlike the language you have been accustomed to all these years. The heart speaks to you in a soft, kind and gentle voice. It never yells out for attention, and gives you a reassuring feeling that you are on the right path or taking the right course of action.

One of the ways in which I know I am communing with my heart is that I notice a radiating and tingling sensation in my chest area which begins to rise through the back of my neck and into my head. I feel my heart speak to me at times through the simplest aspects of life such as the beautiful colors of the morning sunrise or the way in which a Sunday afternoon in autumn looks and feels like. This is your heart talking to you.

A useful exercise to undertake is simply becoming aware and noting in your external environment, what causes your heart to stir with the emotion. Is it a piece of music that no matter many times you listen to it, the music still stirs a response? Is it the feeling you get when someone compliments you on something you have said, something you have done or the way you look? It may be a simple as a thank you that you receive from someone when you help them crossed street or draw a person's attention to the fact that they have dropped some money while they are waiting in queue in front of you?

Whatever it is, take mental notes of these moments rather than dismissing them as pleasant moments. The more you develop this language, the better you are able to know yourself and make decisions that are in harmony with your deepest self. Your heart knows the truth of your being and will reassure you with this knowingness in a soft, silent voice. It is not obtrusive as the mind or the ego screaming for attention. It is silent, pleasant and has no agenda other than the fulfillment of your desires.

Learning to develop a relationship with your heart center may take some practice and also a shift in awareness. Do not be too concerned with attempting to attain anything quickly, for if you try to force the experience you may be met with disappointment. Instead, allow yourself to be immersed with the frequency of *Navigating Life* by becoming better acquainted with that silence and deep inner wisdom, which is continually serving you.

This inner wisdom is available to you and does not take a vacation or breaks. At first many people find the switch from using a logical left brain orientated way of life challenging as we have been accustomed, since early childhood to use logic and reason to shape and create our world.

Females develop their intuitive abilities during this time, which serves them well since they are able to work with both frequencies and energies.

Your heart knows what is right for you. Do not be dissuaded from going deep into your heart with your logical brain, which may step into override this connection.

As you go deeper into your heart, you may become aware of the emotions that were buried long ago. These emotions may take the form of sadness, grief, anger, resentment or other forms of disempowerment, which stops you from leading a life full of passion, enthusiasm and happiness. Do not create more meaning around these emotions by inviting your logical mind to heal these negative states. Instead, just be with the emotion and observe by becoming one with it.

The process of awareness runs deep within your consciousness and this practice of silently witnessing the emotion can do a great deal in order to heal the emotion. If there is a sense of sadness within, then just go to that place within your body where that sadness resides and be with it. When we talk about being with that emotion, it is as though you were treating it by sitting down next to it and merely observe, listen and feel what the emotion expresses. Do not be concerned with trying to heal the emotion or allow the emotion to go away, since doing so will only insight more of the same energy that fuels the emotion into growing stronger and more powerful.

In modern-day culture we feel the need to fix things when they are broken. This way of thinking has continued to shape the way we treat our illnesses and disease. We want to fix that which is broken, yet the heart cannot be fixed in the same manner. The heart yearns to be heard, it seeks to be consoled and nurtured without reason or logic intervening. It is often said that the heart has reasons that reason cannot know. As you become better acquainted with the language of the heart it will serve you in ways that will uplift your spirit and allow you to reconnect with the inner source of your being.

So as you learn to be with this inner source of guidance, you will be offered powerful insights into your deepest self. Honor these insights by stepping into the process and working with the guidance that you have been given. Do not deny nor neglect the inner wisdom as nonsense. Instead come from a place of allowing. Allow the wisdom and possibility of life to reveal itself through your inner being. Observe through silent witnessing by allowing reason and logic to take a back seat.

In order to heal your life and bring peace and joy to your world, you must allow what is to come up and rather than process it, just be with it. Sit and listen with the inner guidance and make a vow to take the journey to the deepest part of yourself. Recall that many of us have buried our emotions deep within the recesses of our hearts. For whatever reason you chose to do this at the time, it is worth turning inward in order to unlock and release this emotional burden and that you deal with it in a compassionate manner.

Each time you honor the deepest wisdom of your heart, you feel a lightness of your body, these are toxic emotions being released as you undertake the healing process. Make a vow by declaring to your inner self that you will dig deep to heal any part of yourself that needs to be healed. Anytime you become aware of any negative emotion, which brings you pain and misery, take action by attending to it with compassion. Be kind and gentle on yourself in the process. You are talking to the little inner child within you, who wants love and affection, not criticism and judgment. Think about the way you would address your children and use the same approach to converse with your inner child.

Chapter Summary:

- The incessant internal dialogue and chatter that takes place in your mind is not the 'real' you – it is merely your mind making up time and space, constructing stories to fit your world.

- Most people listen to the internal chatter taking place in their minds, yet neglect the expression of the heart. The heart has a frequency which is 50,000 times greater than the brain.

- Your heart does not have an agenda or bias like the mind does. It is pure and speaks to you in silent whispers.

- Commune regularly with your heart by going into silence throughout your day. You do not have to devote thirty minutes or more to meditative practice to develop pure awareness.

- Be aware of your predominant thought patterns and observe them. Do not enter into a dialogue with your thoughts – observe and witness them.

- Honor the wisdom offered to you through your heart. Your reaction may be to analyze it with your mind, yet retreating into silence for as little as ten minutes throughout the day allows you to develop a communication channel with your heart center.

- Many people's emotions have been buried deep within their hearts. The deep sadness is longing to be acknowledged. Retreat into your heart by noting through awareness, what your heart wants you to know.

- As you journey into the center of your being, you will discover a fountain of joy and peace which resides within. This is the essence of your true spirit. Allow this part of you to emerge as you replace the old emotions that no longer serve you.

CHAPTER ELEVEN

Navigate Your Emotional Well-being

Be Inspired

"When you are inspired by some great purpose, some extraordinary project, and all your thoughts break their bonds: your mind transcends limitations, your consciousness expands in every direction, and you find yourself in a new, great and wonderful world. Dormant forces, faculties and talents become alive, and you discover yourself to be a greater person by far than you ever dreamed yourself to be."

Patanjali

In his book, The Agony and the Ecstasy, Irving Stone takes the reader on a detailed journey on Michelangelo's life from his early days with the Medici family right through to his detailed sculptures and painting at the Sistine Chapel. The common theme depicted in the book was of an inspired painter and sculpture who lived for his art. Although Michelangelo was supremely talented, he still devoted much of his waking life to developing these talents. He spent numerous hours, even working throughout the night, to dissect cadavers so that he could have a better understanding of the human form. He tirelessly sketched and sculptured the purest Carrara marble, turning blocks of stone into the finest masterpieces the world has known. He once remarked that when sculpturing, the marble took on a life of its own and would tell him how it was to turn out. He was merely the conduit between the marble and the masterpiece revealing itself through him.

Inspiration is the call from your soul to express itself through you. It is no secret that inspired people engage life with every faculty of their being. They are happier, motivated and in love with their passion. They embody their love with every part of their being and ruminate on it every moment they are awake. It literally consumes their life. Inspiration is the expression of creativity and the mind of the universe flowing through you.

And it is not just for artists. If you yearn for direction in your life, inspiration may be calling. Most people do not really know what inspires them. Let us take look at ways you can find inspiration in your life.

While some artists are inspired by nature, others are inspired by humans and their ways of living. We all have different inspiration sources. Some of us need to look within for inspiration, while others have to look outwards. There is actually no golden answer when it comes to finding inspiration and there can be multiple answers for an individual. Nobody can tell you what should or should not inspire you. When I look back at my life, I see that I have been inspired by different things at different times. As a teenager, I was inspired by my favorite band. I wanted to be a musician like them. As times change, our inspirations and role models change.

Focus on what you want now.

What interests and pursuits do you regularly undertake that bring you joy? Do not worry at this stage whether you can derive an income from it. Is it something creative or do you find inspiration in tasks nobody else seems to have time nor patience for?

How do you know that you are inspired by your pursuit and not just happy to be doing it? Well, inspiration is something that brings you deep joy. When you are inspired and pursuing your passion, time stands still.

I find that when I am speaking about my passion in front of audiences, time does stands still and I am lost and absorbed in the moment of my craft. Words just seem to pour forth and I am neither attached nor invested in the exact words that I speak. I have often finished giving a seminar and cannot recall a single thing I have said, despite having rehearsed and planned the topic in advance. I feel joy and bliss radiating from my body when I am present and aware in the moment. I have no desire other than to be the conduit for my thoughts to manifest themselves as words that resonate with my audiences. You may have a similar experience in terms of how inspiration looks and feels to you?

Connect with that feeling of inspiration daily by tuning into its frequency. People who are inspired often comment that they really do not mind whether they are paid or not to pursue their passion. They could work tirelessly for days, weeks or years, yet the common element to their passion is the joy and the fulfillment of them.

There is a well-known passage by Patanjali, who wrote the ancient yoga sutras. The passage reads: *[when] you are inspired by some great purpose, some extraordinary project, and all your thoughts break their bonds: your mind transcends limitations, your consciousness expands in every direction, and you find yourself in a new, great and wonderful world. Dormant forces, faculties and talents become alive, and you discover yourself to be a greater person by far than you ever dreamed yourself to be.*

I have shared this passage with audience members and I am still surprised to discover how deep the meaning of the passage resonates with people.

Patanjali advises us that when we are connected with a deeper purpose, our thoughts transcend their limitations as our consciousness expands and we find ourselves in a new and wonderful world. Our hidden talents become alive as they shine forth and in doing so we discover ourselves to be greater than we ever imagined.

The passage suggests that when you align with a greater force, this is the essence of inspiration. People who are inspired act from a deeper place within. They are not concerned with accolades and recognition from others, they strive for personal satisfaction and a sense of purpose and meaning, which derives from their work.

It is important to understand that inspired people choose to view their work as play and therefore at the end of a working week they have really allowed themselves to play rather than work.

I recall times where I have worked over sixty to seventy hours consistently for weeks, yet as I reflect back I can see that my work was an opportunity to play. And whilst tiredness and fatigue are part of the process, the opportunity to play at something you are passionate and inspired to do far outweighs turning up to a nine to five job which you dislike.

So how do you know that you are inspired? What does inspiration look like when you become aligned with this faculty?

You are inspired when you identify with the following characteristics:

- You love what you do
- You cannot wait to wake up in the morning to pursue your passion.
- Time seems to stand still when you are pursuing your passion.
- You are energized and full of life when pursuing your passion.
- It does not matter that you are not getting paid since you gain a great deal from your work.
- Being creative is an opportunity to display and reveal your hidden talents.
- So absorbed in your work, you are unaware of anything else in your life.
- You are continually looking for new ways to improve upon the work that you do.
- You approach your passion with a sense of humility and gratitude.
- You feel an inner sense of peace and security when pursuing your passion.
- You might notice the feelings of anxiety and tension when you go for long periods without pursuing your passion.

- You love the satisfaction it brings you if others complement you on your work – you do not necessarily seek approval from others.

It is obvious from the characteristics listed above that those pursuing their passion do so with a level of inspiration, which is beyond the call of duty. Inspired people work from inside out, rather than requiring continual motivation.

There is often some confusion between inspiration and motivation. Given the list of characteristics above, you can clearly see that an inspired person does not require motivation. However, people who require motivation need an external source to keep them progressing along their path. A good example of looking at motivation might suggest that in order to motivate someone you would have a hand on their back, nudging them forward. When you take your hand away, the person is less inclined to stay motivated.

Inspired people are their own motivators. They do not need the motivation from an external source in order to keep them inspired. The source of their inspiration comes from a deep place within. Inspired people are deeply aware of the inner source of their inspiration, which emanates and creates the passion and enthusiasm that they feel toward their work and purpose.

Inspired Purpose

Those who are inspired find meaning and purpose to their work. They view their purpose as a calling rather than a job or career. Because of this they operate from a higher frequency, allowing the source of their inspiration to flow unimpeded through every cell of their body.

You will also be pleased to know that inspiration, because of its higher frequency acts on the mind and body, thus allowing the individual to thrive at eight different states. You might call this state a higher vibrational frequency, which is the flow of the creative intelligence that we all have access to. I have purposely called this section of the chapter *Inspired Purpose* because I believe that they are mutually dependent upon one another. That is when you are pursuing your purpose in life there is no other way of being other than inspired.

It is rare to find someone who is deeply passionate, enthusiastic and pursuing their purpose in life who is not inspired to create their reality. For this reason I have included inspiration as a blueprint for *Navigating Life*, because I believe that the world needs more inspired leaders to share their vision with humanity. Your vision and purpose is a gift from the universe. You are the representation of the creative universal intelligence and therefore your goals, your vision and your purpose is an extension of the universe allowing itself to create through you.

The word universe simply means, "one song," which highlights the unification of time space and matter all coexisting together at the precise moment of creation. What this means to you is that as a creative expression of this one song, you have been given that same verse in which to create and paint your masterpiece. That masterpiece is your gift and your passion and in order to fulfill that passion and purpose, the universe has also given you inspiration in which to realize the creative process.

Let us take a look at some ways in which you can become inspired and create the future that you wish to see. Do not mistake your past as a gauge or grounds from which to create your future anew. For back then you were not living with inspiration, operating from motivation or perspiration. These are lower states of frequencies that are not imbued with one important ingredient - love.

Life and inspiration also coexist together since the universe is also built on a life energy and frequency. When you connect and align with this frequency and energy of love, you tap into the language of the universe and become the expression of that life energy. Your purpose becomes your passion and you have no other way than to love your work and purpose.

We conclude that the universal formula for inspiration looks like the following:

Purpose + Love + Passion = **Inspiration**

Your purpose when aligned with the highest frequency of love combines with passion equals inspiration. What this means is that in order to acquire and maintain inspiration for what you do, allow your work to become your purpose and then subsequently match that with passion and love and you have no other avenue than to become inspired.

Before we reflect on the ways in which to become inspired, take a moment and think about your current circumstances. Reflect on your current job, whether that is your career, your calling or merely a means to make ends meet to pay the bills. If you are studying, is the course of your studies allowing you to edge closer toward pursuing your purpose?

If what you are currently pursuing right now is in the area of what you are passionate about and approached with enthusiasm and love, then inevitably you are inspired or draw inspiration from this pursuit. If you are pursuing a job or a course of study merely because you do not know what you are passionate about or what you love, that is fine as long as you continue searching for something that resonates with your inner being.

The famous mythologist, writer and lecturer Joseph Campbell said, *follow your bliss and the universe will open doors for you where there were only walls.* I recall first reading this passage, it struck a chord with me at the time as I was searching for my purpose and passion in life. Joseph Campbell reminds us that when pursuing our passion and purpose with intent, vigor and meaning the universe aligns to bring you the right people, circumstances, events and situations in order to realize your dream and vision.

I believe that Joseph Campbell is guiding us to pursue our passion and purpose by alluding to the "walls" signifying the dead ends and roadblocks which once prevented us from being inspired. Following your bliss allows you to access that deep wisdom of creativity and knowledge that is self-contained in every person. In order to pursue your passion and live from a place of inspiration it is essential that you awaken the creative intelligence within you.

On the coming pages I have listed some ideas to help you become inspired. Chances are that you already know what you are passionate about and enjoy doing, yet you may feel inadequate about taking your creativity and genius out into the world. This is quite common for people starting out since they have not had the experience of creating and sharing their passion with others.

I suggest you start in a small way, and it could be as simple as writing a weekly blog in which you share your thoughts and creative expression with other people. Note the responses that you get from those visiting your site and become attuned to what people are commenting about. Typically when you begin to share your creativity with others, your audience will naturally respond by telling you what they would like to see. Take this on board by adapting your own style to suit your audience.

This may be true of anything suited towards your passion and purpose. Along the way as you produce a product or service, people will naturally gravitate toward your work by simultaneously giving you clues and suggestions as to their current problems. Listen and be attentive to what your audience is telling you and respond with your take on solving their problem.

Ideas to help you become inspired

If you still are unable to find your source of inspiration, try these:

- Read biographies of successful or great people.
- Travel and visit another cultures. Familiarize yourself with the local people.
- Go to photography exhibitions and see the beauty captured in images. See past the photos and feel what the artist is attempting to capture.
- Go to the beach and enjoy a quiet walk. This will give you time to reflect on your inner self.
- Go to new restaurants and try different types of food. Eat something that you have never tasted before. Many world-class chefs get their inspiration this way.
- Go out with friends and have a hearty chat over a long coffee break.

- Read novels about people who have been inspired to create masterpieces. (Irving Stone's book on Michelangelo certainly stirred a passion within me.)

- Listen to a new kind of music. Select a new genre and enjoy it.

- Teach other people. Impart your knowledge. This will give you happiness.

It is important to create a space in your daily life to become open to inspiration. If you currently work in a job or career that is not your purpose and passion, it is worth spending some time in your day engaging with your passion. Just because you cannot derive an income from it at this stage does not mean not devoting your time and attention toward becoming proficient and an expert in your area. Author Malcolm Gladwell suggests that in order to be world class in your chosen field, you must spend the equivalent of 10,000 hours practicing and harnessing your craft.

The notable key toward inspiration is that it will not come looking for you while you are sitting around waiting for it to show up. One needs to be engaged, pursuing something that they have an interest for and enjoy doing. This may later transform itself into inspiration as you slowly find yourself doing more of it. Do not be concerned with seeking out inspiration and applying it to your current circumstances.

Pursue excellence with vigor and enthusiasm and success and passion will naturally follow. Do not be too anxious with the end result, engage yourself in the journey by being engaged in the present moment when pursuing your passion.

Lastly, become inspired. Talk to people by networking and socializing with like-minded individuals. The more you share your passion and enthusiasm about your work with others, the more you will learn and gain from them. Connecting with others who are interested in your area of interest allows you to meet different people and learn new things from them.

Ultimately, the more you share your knowledge, wisdom, passion and enthusiasm toward your work with others; the more inclined people are to respond with the same level of enthusiasm toward your shared interest.

Chapter Summary:

- Inspiration is a calling from your soul to express your talents and gifts to the world.

- The key to becoming inspired is taking what you are passionate about right now and pursuing that with purpose and meaning.

- The obvious signs of inspiration are; joy, passion, enthusiasm, love, dedication, purpose, meaning, creativity, desire, fulfillment and satisfaction.

- Inspiration has a frequency that is greater than motivation. It engages your mind body and spirit.

- The formula for inspiration combines the following aspects; Purpose + Love + Passion = Inspiration.

- Love is an essential ingredient when you are inspired since your purpose comes from a deeper place within your heart.

- Joseph Campbell talks about following your bliss and the universe opening doors were there were once walls. He reminds us about the need to pursue our passion and become inspired to be of service to others.

- Attend to your purpose and passion on a daily basis by making room for it in your life, whether it is a small portion of your day or greater – the more you make time for it, the greater it will serve you.

CHAPTER TWELVE

Navigate Your Emotional Well-being

Let Go of Things Which Do not Serve You

"Holding on to anger is like grasping a hot coal with the intent of throwing it at someone else; you are the one who gets burned."

Buddha

We spend so much of our life forming attachments to things, people, places, thoughts and emotions that our lives become overburdened with trivial things that really do not matter. Suffering stems from holding onto things which do not serve us – yet in a strange way, it seems comforting and familiar to hold onto these things for fear that they will not be replaced or will be gone from our lives if we let go. The truth of the matter is the universe immediately fills the space in your life when you make a conscious decision to let go of that which does not serve you.

Letting go of things that do not serve you is as simple as dropping the thoughts, the emotion or circumstance that takes up residency within you. There is another way of looking at it, much like the toys you used to play with when you were a child. As an adult they no longer serve you the same way as they did when you are a child. You might even call many of the attachments that you had toward certain aspects of your early life, which also have dropped away to make way for new things.

Life offers you the same lifeline by encouraging you to let go of anything which is taxing you mentally, emotionally, physically and spiritually.

Take an inventory of your current circumstances and investigate those areas which cause you to be unhappy and unfulfilled. They might be toxic or draining relationships. Invariably these relationships drain you and provide no personal growth for either party. Yet we find evidence to substantiate the relationship in our life. These may include innumerable reasons, when at the essence of it all, we continue to suffer within.

Reflect on those relationships that draw energy away from you and leave you feeling empty inside and uninspired. How will you know that these relationships exist in your life? One sure way is to look to your physiology and note how you feel on the occasions you meet with these people. Is there a sense of being unfulfilled that arises when you meet with such people? Rather than immediately severing your ties with such individuals, you might slowly distance yourself from them by not accepting invitations to social gatherings. Slowly over time you will find yourself in a happier place by attracting those people whom you wish to spend your time with. You must also become that, which you wish to attract.

If you desire to have more love, honest and trustworthy connections in your life, then it stands to reason that you must also become the embodiment of those qualities and values yourself. Friendships and connections can only be formed by like-minded individuals who vibrate on the same frequency. It does not matter that you have different personalities or interests. What matters is that to have the same outlook on life and value the integrity of close and fulfilling connections.

As you begin to pursue fulfilling and sustainable relationships, you will notice that you align yourself with things that really matter. You will become aware of things that are important as you allow room and space for them in your life. You will be naturally drawn and inclined toward such circumstances since they provide you with a sense of joy, peace and fulfillment. It is it similar to when you undertake a health and fitness regime where you no longer eat toxic foods, instead gravitating towards nutritious and healthy food choices. You might also undertake physical exercise during this period and become aware of how well you feel as you progress along your journey.

Letting go of things which do not serve you also brings you the same sense of satisfaction. You will notice the inner reward that comes to you when you are doing things which bring you happiness and joy, that you will no longer attract toxic or negative situations. This is also the case with your *Health and Well-being* program—your mind and body become attuned to higher states of wellness and they no longer require destructive or toxic habits to provide the same sense of fulfillment that they once did.

Resist the urge to obsess about insignificant circumstances, things or events which no longer serve you. Check-in with yourself by asking the previously given questions:

Navigating Life empowers you to make decisions that are in harmony with your deepest self; the essence of who you truly are. In the earlier chapter we spoke about the difference between the *Parked* and *Navigating* states.

Those who remain *Parked* also remained stagnant and incomplete in unfulfilling relationships. They feel a sense of duty and obligation to remain in a relationship or connection that does not serve their well-being. Despite their best intentions not to hurt the other person by cutting the connection, they are in fact doing more harm than good both to themselves and the other party by staying in a relationship which does not serve either party, nor the universe. Allow me to preface this by also saying that it takes a great deal of courage and self-awareness to identify the truth.

Honor yourself by making decisions that are in alignment and in harmony with the truth of who you are. Far too many people live out of a sense of duty and obligation to others, while simultaneously depriving themselves of their own power. This ultimately deprives real connection between others, since you are not being your authentic self.

One of the greatest misconceptions in our modern era is the sense of lack that many people feel toward attaining goodness in their life.

For this reason many people's decisions come from a place of lack which is shrouded in fear. The fear denotes the fear of the unknown, the uncertain element of what life brings if and when you let go of that which does not serve you.

Recall earlier we spoke about the universe coming to your rescue by filling a space in your life. The analogy in your life may be akin to thoughts that no longer serve you, outdated relationships or things which no longer take precedent in your life. The universe and its creative energy is aware of these subtle changes within your life, because you are an expression of universal intelligence and therefore it knows best how to attend to your needs. Your job is to merely play your part in co-creating the circumstances of your life and leave the how-to process up to the universe. This involves a level of detachment and surrender and also faith that all your needs will be met, but only when you stand back and allow the process to unfold.

The best way to step into your power and reclaim your sense of entitlement within the framework of the cosmos is to start small. Make decisions which are within your comfort zone and watch the process unfold. The beauty of this is that as you begin to see evidence of life coming to your aid, you will naturally develop your belief muscle and in no time you will be making bigger decisions that are in harmony with your deepest desires. An example of starting small might include creating an intention to let go of personal belongings that no longer serve you. A good place to start may be any personal belongings you have not used in the last three to six months. Make a personal statement to yourself and the universe that you will be guided toward passing on these items to people or charities that are in need of these donations. Make a silent declaration to yourself and to the universe for guidance on how and when these items should be released.

Naturally, as you make this declaration the creative universal intelligence will guide you toward the right people that are in need of your items. You may feel a sudden impulse toward giving your items to a certain charity or alternatively an ad may appear in your letterbox advertising for second-hand items. Whatever way the universe decides is best to re-purpose your belongings will be made known to you at the right time, when and if your intentions are correctly aligned with the gift of giving.

The universe operates in mysterious ways that are unbeknownst to our mortal minds. We tend to think in linear patterns and in doing so, disallow a great deal of the mystery and synchronicities to eventuate. The universe specializes in the unknown and operates on a multidimensional level. This means that circumstances and events will transpire, not according to your own timeframe. Be open and receptive to the unknown by creating a space in your life for these occurrences.

Besides, who wants to live a boring and dull life? I often hear people talking about how boring and mundane their lives have become as all they seem to be doing is carrying out the same tasks from day to day. Many of these same people, when prompted do not believe in mysteries and synchronicities and so miss out on the infinite possibilities that are available to them at the moment they relinquish and surrender the notion of how life should unfold.

When you live life from this perspective, you begin to see each situation as a mystery and with synchronicity. Rather than becoming attached to your own agenda, that governs the timing of how things should play out in your life; you come from a place of allowing which is seeded in infinite possibilities. Recall earlier that life does not know what it will become until it reveals itself.

There are a number of possibilities for events and circumstances to unfold and they can only do so once we detach both mentally and emotionally from the situation. Instead, if you surrender control by allowing yourself to be grateful for whatever shows up in your life, you will find joy, peace and fulfillment in everything that you co-create with universal energy.

The challenge for many people is learning to detach from this essence of how life should unfold. Many find it challenging and almost impossible to believe that something greater than us actually knows what is best for you. This limited way of thinking prevents you from mastering the real lessons of life, one of which is detachment.

Detachment does not mean apathy, in fact quite the opposite. Detachment implies that we handover the process of life to a greater force that knows best on how to attend to our needs and wants. We stand in a place of firm understanding and knowledge that everything we truly want and need will be delivered to us once we surrender control and allow our egoistic nature to stand idle.

Practicing Detachment

The practice of detachment may be challenging initially since the mind is drawn to habitually analyzing events and situations. You may find that as you allow detachment to work for you, your mind will intervene by creating a story and a running analysis of the inherent flaws of detachment. Despite this, I suggest you stick with it and every time you find yourself clinging to a thought, an emotion, a person or situation, merely let it go.

The Buddha said *holding on to anger is like grasping a hot coal with the intent of hrowing it at someone else; you are the one who gets burned.* With that in mind, we can take this teaching further and relate it to detachment by dropping the hot coal when an unwanted thought or circumstance presents itself in our life. Tara Brach in her book, *True Refuge,* cites the work of brain scientist Jill Bolte Taylor who suggests that the average lifespan of an emotion to move through the nervous system is one and a half minutes. Knowing this releases the burden that we need to carry our emotional attachments longer than need be.

Reflect for a moment and write down any thoughts, beliefs or emotions, whether positive or negative, that you have held on to for a long time. Examine your list and ask yourself the following question: *How does this thought, belief or emotion serve me?* If you are repeatedly playing out a negative thought, how does that thought actually serve you? You might say it allows me to feel assured that thinking negative thoughts takes the burden off positive expectations of things being better. Ultimately we do not want to be let down and so we attach ourselves to toxic or negative thoughts. When life shows us evidence of this negativity, we are in a position to substantiate the thoughts since reality has proven so.

This is certainly not the way to live your life as you remain in a *Parked* state in relation to your thoughts that drive your words and actions. Through conscious self-awareness, you are able to highlight these unwanted thought patterns and examine them so as they do not occupy space in your mind. In order to practice detachment, you must be routinely aware of any thought, emotion or behavior that you entertain. So awareness is the first step toward detachment.

As you begin to become better at observing your thoughts, emotions and actions, you are in a better position to intercede by creating new and empowering thoughts and actions. There is no need to analyze your inner world for in doing so you give more energy and subsequently your mind creates an enriching story around this. As we discussed in previous chapters, becoming the silent witness or the observer is enough to draw your awareness to the situation. As soon as you allow consciousness to step in, you have taken the first step toward releasing the thought, belief or emotion.

Allow me to preface this by suggesting that this must become a constant process for your mind will cling to these scenarios, particularly if you entertain them over the years. So let us take a quick look at the process of detachment:

- Allow consciousness to observe through Mindfulness and silently witness the thought, belief or emotion.

- Do not create a story around this but merely be with it.

- Avoid trying to change or fix the thought, belief or emotion as doing so will give it more energy.

- Ask yourself the question, how do these thoughts, belief and emotions serve me?

- Refuse to get drawn in to mind games, and like a piece of hot coal drop anything that does not serve you.

- Become aware of any sensations within your body and notice where they reside. Notice the intensity and the feelings that they offer you.

If you practice detachment, over time, you will find yourself in a more peaceful and tranquil state.

I have found that the more I detach from the outcomes, the more I come from a place of allowing life to reveal itself in the best possible way. I remove my ego and my preconceived perceptions and history from playing out and deciding my future. The more you learn to detach, the more life takes on a new meaning and there is a sense of awe and wonder.

Do not be hard on yourself if you initially discover the process to be more challenging than what it is worth. Stick with it and I can assure you that in due course you will arrive at a place in your mind and heart that is free of anxiety, fear and worry.

Chapter Summary:

- Take inventory of things which do not bring you joy and remove them from your life.

- The universe will fill a space in your life when you make room for it. Your mind and heart are spaces that will be filled with goodness.

- Align yourself with things that really matter. Stop obsessing about small things which consume your time and energy.

- Be ruthless with pursuing that which resonates with your deepest self – insist on it.

- Do not hold onto things for fear or fear of the unknown.

- Start small and get rid of clutter and unwanted things, people and circumstances.

- Attend to meaningful relationships in your life and remove yourself from people who do not inspire you to become better.

- Be open and receptive to the unknown aspects of life – make room for mystery since this is the basis for living in wonder and awe.

- Learn to detach from thoughts, beliefs and emotions which do not serve you anymore. Simply drop them like a hot piece of coal.

- Go through the six step process of detachment to free yourself from the hold of anxiety, fear and worry.

- Be kind and gentle on yourself as you learn detachment. It is natural that you will slip-up from time to time.

CHAPTER THIRTEEN

Navigate Your Emotional Well-being

Honor and Respect Yourself
Honor Your Feelings

"We have to dare to be ourselves, however frightening or strange that self may prove to be."

May Sarton

The sixth blueprint for *Navigating Life* asks that you honor and respect yourself as a means of standing in your own power. Honoring yourself means inviting the deepest part of your authentic self to come forth as an expression of the real you. Too many people hide behind a veil which keeps them trapped mentally, emotionally and physically reliving situations that are neither desirable or wanted in their life.

They feel helpless and stuck unable to *Navigate* toward a more empowering state. This can become a vicious cycle in which negative mental and emotional states are played out in one's life, so that you begin to think that this is normal. Many people buy into this way of life, believing they are a product of their environment and therefore unable to change or create the circumstances of their life. You are more than your thoughts about yourself or any situation outside of you. Any untoward thought occurring within your mind does so because you entertain it regularly by giving it energy; it grows and spreads its tentacles into larger dominant thoughts. You have the power to break out of this cycle at your choosing by stepping into your own power and reclaiming your life.

So how do you honor yourself? To honor yourself means to honor the deepest part of you by owning and stepping into your own power. *Navigating Life* means taking ownership of your emotions—not only when they are positive and empowering emotions, but also when they are undesirable. These emotions may include rage, anger, grief, sadness or any lower emotional states. You are being invited to examine an emotion and accept it as an aspect of your wholeness rather than shove it deeper into your unconscious mind or deny it.

On the other hand people who deny their emotional nature remain *Parked* and stagnant in their life, as the emotion has the potential to dominate their life. Your emotions will always win since they are absolute and you cannot negotiate with strong emotions, especially if they have been present since childhood.

What are your emotions trying to teach you? This is the way to reframe it in your mind. Rather than looking at the emotion as unwanted because it feels unwelcoming, ask yourself a simple question, *what might this emotion be asking of me?* Or another way of looking at it might be, *who will I become when I honor this emotion by reclaiming my power?* Inevitably the emotion allows us to deal with a hidden part of ourselves that may be unconscious and connected to our earlier life as children.

I have dealt with many of these unconscious emotions which have surfaced at various stages of my life. Rather than run away from them and place them deeper into the unconscious self, I chose to look at them with an open heart and open mind. I chose to deal with them with an unbiased perspective that perhaps I may have gained vital wisdom about a part of me that I may have neglected or suppressed. When I approached the situation from this mindset, I allowed my emotions to take center stage and freely express anything they were inviting me to understand.

As children grow up they are largely influenced by their parents and people of authority. Our greatest learning and understanding take place in those formative years between our birth and the ages of six to seven years. My upbringing was no different to other children; I had a loving home and was cared and nurtured for by wonderful parents who made a new life in this country, having immigrated from abroad. Both worked hard to provide for me and my two sisters. My father worked hard and we were never denied anything as children. Love was abundant, thanks to a sweet and caring mother who made sure our needs were met.

Being the only male among my siblings, my relationship with my father was at times strenuous, especially as I approached my teenage years. Since he was brought up in a very disciplined home himself, my upbringing and discipline was routinely matched with what he observed as a child growing up in a poor family. My father was stern and insisted on perfection and the best from me. This was hard to achieve as a child since nothing I could do matched his level of expectation – there was always more one could do he would quip.

Evidently, later in my life, I adopted the same attitude toward myself and insisted on perfection in everything I did. I was equally hard and stern with myself as he was, since I was modeling his behavior toward me. I had taken on his persona and adapted it to suit my needs – yet they were not how I envisaged myself to be. Underneath that exterior of toughness was a shy and introverted male who was emotionally sensitive. I still recall back then, the anxiety that flooded my body when my father yelled at me for something I had done. That same feeling still resonated with me into my adult years and I avoided confrontation with anyone at all costs.

However bad I believed things to be at the time, I am certain there was an emotional aspect that I denied or even buried deep for fear of allowing myself to be weak or inferior. I recall during my post teenage years the thoughts of unworthiness that dominated my mental landscape; I felt incapable and unworthy of goodness since I had accepted that as my story as a child. It was only through self-examination that I learned these were aspects of me that I denied, fearing that if I faced them, I would no longer accept and like the person who was behind all that.

Nonetheless, my greatest wisdom was gained when I accepted all my flaws, failures and shortcomings, while accepting that I was more than all these things I had labeled myself to be. Behind these facades was a shining light, much like the moon we spoke about earlier. Sure at times, it might be obscured by the light of the sun, but the moon still remains the moon in all its glory. It is similar to the intimate relationship you share with your partner or husband/wife. You might discover a part of their character or nature that you do not like initially, but as time passes, you learn that they are more than these trivial set of flaws and defects and you learn to love and accept them even more. This is what it means to own and accept every part of you.

Navigating your emotional well-being invites you to tend to your thoughts and emotions. Consider who you are becoming with the thoughts and emotions that you carry with you? We become the sum of our thoughts, which drive our emotional state; therefore what you entertain on a day-to-day basis is expressed through you. You are what you repeatedly think about.

Before long their emotional well-being is compromised, as like an iceberg, 80% of it remains submerged under the water. It is often a little too late to attend to one's emotional well-being since the emotions have been repressed for far too long and begin to express themselves physiologically through the body as pain, illness or disease.

By honoring and respecting yourself, you are Navigating your emotional well-being by honoring your thoughts and emotions. As you become better at observing your thoughts, they have less of an impact on you as you become less inclined to identify with them and give them energy. You begin to understand that you are not the sum of your thoughts and that thoughts are happening to you, rather than taking ownership of the thoughts.

Self-Worth

Low self-esteem may have arisen in one's life for a number of reasons, although it is normally a call to reconnect and reawaken your true and authentic self. Low self-esteem is merely a mental and emotional state you wish to avoid attaching yourself to. For many people low self-worth becomes a condition of reality, since they have identified with this persona for many years. They inevitably take on this role as being the truth. Subsequently, low self-worth manifests itself in various forms to include relationships, family, finances and career. Low self-esteem is like driving a car with the handbrake on. You may wonder why you are not able to go any faster and yet for some reason you intuitively know that this is possible. Something does not make sense although you are unaware of what is the cause of the problem.

So how does one develop self-worth? It begins at the level of the mind by being attentive to your thought process. Now this does not mean analyzing every thought that enters your mind, yet noticing the themes of your thoughts is a positive step in the right direction. *Are your thoughts self-sabotaging or self-deprecating? Do you put yourself down when things do not go your way? Do you insist on perfection in everything you do?* These types of thoughts may be connected to low self-esteem since the individual turns on him or herself rather than embracing their uniqueness.

As you attend to your thoughts, which may include being in silence throughout the day, you will naturally find that these predominant thoughts take a back seat ride instead of dominating your mental landscape. It is as though you have turned down the volume on these incessant thoughts and taken a step back from identifying with them as the essence of your being. Naturally, inner peace and harmony emerges to connect with your mind and heart, since these two aspects are always present within you, though they may have been denied expression in the past.

Personal Growth

Regular personal growth is the basis for honoring and respecting yourself. It is a continuing process for those wishing to *Navigate Life*. Personal growth is an important aspect of *Navigating Life*. This is because we attend to our mental, emotional and spiritual well-being. Our lives become the embodiment of joy and fulfillment as we harness our true potential, whilst acknowledging and attending to the deepest part of our nature.

Regular personal growth simply means noticing and becoming aware of thought patterns or toxic emotions and attending to them through self-examination. The point of this process is to challenge the basis to your thoughts and emotions. *Are these thoughts the real you? Who would you be without these thoughts?* So as we undertake the journey of personal growth, we invest in our self-worth by attending to our inner world which is naturally reflected in the external world.

Change is difficult at the best of times, although it does not have to be intimidating or unapproachable. The reason that we fear change is for a variety of reasons. Although primarily, we fear the unknown, we fear and may dislike what emerges once we undertake the change process. That should not be a deterrent to stop you from pursuing personal growth on regular basis. Fearing the unknown or what may emerge is only compounding the problem, for what you fear will consume your life. One needs to step into the unknown and trust that whatever emerges is likely to be for your highest good.

What are ways you can pursue regular personal growth? For starters, begin to notice your predominant thoughts. **Be aware of what you think about and entertain on a regular basis.** Notice the theme of the thoughts, but do not attach yourself to the thoughts. Do not become invested in them through regular internal dialogue. Thoughts are thoughts that come and go from your mind, much like those waves that wash into the shoreline. Becoming invested with your thoughts is akin to wishing that like the waves, they peacefully and serenely wash in.

You also have internal and external influences acting on you, driving your thought process. Being aware of these influences allows you to *Navigate Life* by becoming attuned to your dominant thought patterns. Understanding what you often entertain as thoughts puts you in a powerful position to become self-aware and ultimately attend to these thoughts by giving them less attention than they deserve.

Personal growth invites you to become self-aware and conscious of your thought patterns while questioning the validity of those thoughts. For example if you have self-destructive thoughts about your inability to lose weight, you set yourself up for future failure by programming your subconscious mind toward the realization of those thoughts. If you wish to question these thoughts through self-examination, you would see that these thoughts are indeed invalid and that there is no basis to these thoughts.

I recall a prominent mind-power motivational speaker inviting audience members to contemplate the following question: *If you attach yourself to your thoughts and believe you are your thoughts, what will you think next?* The point he was making with this exercise is that thoughts come and go and change, so therefore to become invested and single out any particular thought would be meaningless. Being attentive to your thoughts is a great step toward changing your thoughts, since you are now consciously aware of thoughts taking place in your mind.

Honoring and respecting yourself also invites you to weed out any thoughts that are not in harmony with the truth of who you are. As the saying suggests, allowing destructive thoughts to occupy space in your mind is like having a bad tenant live in your house rent-free. You are doing the same when you entertain and feed on destructive thoughts.

There are numerous methods that people use to weed out destructive thoughts. These include observing and questioning their thoughts. Observing our thoughts allows us to witness the thoughts without attaching ourself to the story they create.

An exercise that was used earlier in the book asked you to close your eyes and imagine a scenario being played out in your mind. In undertaking this exercise, you would have suspended narrating the story in your mind while your imagination was doing the work. Yet in reality the mind likes to create a story, attaching itself to the thoughts that it frequently entertains.

I have found over the years that by understanding the nature of my thoughts, allowed me to become aware of what I entertain my mind with. In doing so I examined and questioned these thoughts so that ultimately the volume was turned down on them. The way I framed it in my mind was by using the following mind exercise:

I imagine that my thoughts were a monkey that was trying to get my attention by screaming and yelling. At first I would succumb to the monkey by paying it attention. Yet the more I did so the greater the intensity of the thoughts emerged. So instead of giving the thoughts attention, I simply began to notice the thoughts while moving my awareness to something else. The mind is like a monkey, or "monkey mind,"—always agitated and looking for attention. When you draw you attention away from the thoughts coming in, you are giving less thought to the monkey. In this way the monkey may be viewed as sitting under a tree eating bananas instead of being agitated trying to get your attention (thoughts).

You may wish to create your own mental screenplay based on thoughts, which work for you. There is no right or wrong method as long as you stay diligent toward weeding out the thoughts that do not serve you. Like a pendulum swinging out of control, in time and with enough practice and patience, the pendulum finally slows down representing your destructive thoughts until it is barely noticeable.

Chapter Summary:

- Honor your feelings – the deepest part of you.

- Do not deny your shadows, irrespective of why you might label them – good or bad. They are inviting you to accept your wholeness.

- Who are you becoming with the thoughts and emotions you entertain? Attend to them if they are not who you want to be.

- Develop self-esteem. Accept yourself and reclaim any disowned parts of yourself. You are more than what you think about yourself.

- Make personal growth a regular occurrence in your life. Develop time and patience toward understanding who you are and why you are 'who you are'.

- Be attuned to your inner self-talk and weed out negative or self-defeating inner dialogue which does not allow you to become who you wish to be.

- Stand for what you believe in – maintain your conviction that you will accept nothing less than what you deserve.

- Do not become invested with your thoughts by accepting them as the truth. Your thoughts come and go, so clinging to them is useless and futile. You are more than the sum of your thoughts.

CHAPTER FOURTEEN

Navigate Your Emotional Well-being

Forgive and Heal the Past

"You do not see the world as it is. You see it as you are."

Anais Anin

In order to *Navigate Life* and the life of happiness, joy and fulfillment, one must learn to heal any aspect of their past which they are resistant to.

Your resistance to "what is" or "what was" will continue to be the source of your suffering as long as you carry the pain and hurt within you. Many people find it difficult to forgive for a multitude of reasons but chiefly because they feel weakened or vulnerable if and when they decide to forgive. Coming to terms with forgiving the past may be a painstaking process for many, since they feel that in doing so they diminish the pain and suffering that they experienced at the time. Owning your pain and suffering by carrying it through life is one way of remaining *Parked*, since you become a slave to the past by drawing on these memories and experiences—these only serve to remind you that you were victimized.

In this chapter I offer you an alternative perspective on what forgiving and healing the past means. Forgiving and healing the past is about your journey toward freedom and happiness. It is about releasing the burden of hanging onto an event or situation that occurred many years ago in the hope of living a richer and more authentic life, unburdened by painful memories. Recognizing that you may have stuffed down a painful memory is the first step toward healing and reclaiming the past. What we are talking about here is a total acceptance of the past and not being shameful or embarrassed of what occurred.

Oftentimes, people feel victimized by their experience and in doing so take ownership of their hurt by carrying it around like a suitcase. This permits them to feel sad, depressed, and angry or whatever negative state you wish to add. But as you know, victims never heal and if you wish to carry the title of being the most coveted victim in the world, I can assure you that no one will award you that prize as a trophy. Only you have the ability to take responsibility and ownership of the way in which you respond to the past.

It is worth noting that healing and forgiving the past does not deny you the hurt that was experienced at the time. Rather you are choosing not to carry that experience into the present moment and into the future.

You have a choice whether you wish to heal the pain or choose to be right You cannot have it both ways, for life will assuredly acknowledge you either way. Forgiving and healing the past is not an easy process and can only be approached with an open heart and mind. You must be willing to surrender and let go of the pain which you have owned and held so close to you, pain that has become your identity.

So the first step in forgiving and healing the past is surrender. You surrender to the truth that you are prepared to heal the trauma you carry. There is no denying that the healing process may be painful, since it reignites many painful emotions. Therefore, you must approach the healing and forgiving process with a compassionate heart. As covered in previous chapters, the process of detaching from thoughts and emotions allows you to see the 'what is' within each moment. Approaching your forgiveness toward healing the past should also be met with the same detachment and compassion. As your emotions surface and reignites, you may be forced to change and label these emotions, this is not what the healing process is all about.

Healing means accepting, regardless of whether the experience or situation was good or bad. Healing does not mean labeling or judging the experience, for in doing so it disallows you from letting go of any painful emotions. Kindness and compassion towards oneself is of the utmost importance in order to free yourself from the painful memories that keep you trapped in the past.

The past is all but a figment of your imagination. To bring it into the present moment means that you miss out on the beauty and splendor of what this moment has to offer. Your perceptions and experience are being expressed from the past in order to shape and create your present moment experience. The mind is adept at drawing on historical events in order to decide how to give meaning to the current moment. This comes at a price however. The price is that you are not fully awake and aware to your present moment, since you are referencing the past in order to shape the NOW, which ultimately creates the future.

For example, if you have been emotionally abused in previous intimate relationships, then you have created a thought memory and emotional association around this experience. You have painted onto your mental canvas the truth that intimate relationships ultimately lead to emotional abuse. You will be drawn to find evidence of this in each new relationship. Surprisingly, it only takes **one** positive experience with a partner to prove this incorrect. Your past conditioning has perpetuated an experience which has proved true for you and thus perceives it as accurate. **What we fail to recognize is that we form a perception of reality rather than the truth**.

Make it your priority to let go of things, people and circumstances that you have found difficult to forgive. Start small and have no expectation of yourself, other than to find peace. Your motive should be based on your own self-interest and to be at peace with any emotion that remains bound to the past. People who live in the past like to re-live and play out their story. They feel that without their story they would be left empty inside. Their story creates an illusion since they identify with it as being real. You are more than your stories, whether they are based in a positive or negative experience. These are constructs of your mind which allow you to feel something that you are not. By dropping the storyline that you have held for so long, you allow the truth of who you really are emerge. You are an eternal being, one that is not bound by labels and stories, such as those that you commit to yourself.

When you approach life from this perspective, you see that the illusions that you created serve your purpose; to feel safe behind this veil. However, this is not the real you.

There comes a point in your life when you must drop the facade in order to acknowledge your hurt and pain. Stuffing down the pain will only allow it to magnify since you are feeding that which needs to grow. You are giving it importance and life by telling it that it is important and willingly become the victim. It is like taking in a wounded dove and nurturing it for some time, only to discover that you have grown attached to the bird. Despite it being healed, you cling to it in the fear by letting it go you will be sad and empty inside.

The dove was born to fly and roam. By holding onto the belief of this false self, it keeps you trapped in the past, rather than being fully alive and awake to the present moment. Those who are not alive to the present moment will find any excuse to substantiate their situation, since reconciling the past is far more painful than acknowledging the truth. But why live this way? Why show up for life full of luggage hoping to add to your suitcase as you go along? Your luggage is full enough and needs to be emptied of your sorrows and pain in order to lighten the load.

Peace and joy can only be found in the present moment. You have probably witnessed this when you hoped for something or someone to make you feel better. That is because you placed your happiness in some future event or thing hoping that it would heal those parts of you that were in pain. No-thing, person or circumstance will bring you happiness and fulfillment, and this is for a number of reasons. Firstly, you are wishing for something outside of you that is already there, yet fail to acknowledge it. It is like magicians performing their illusion right before your eyes, only later to reveal their secret. You discover that the illusion was not magic after all. It was just trickery of the mind as your awareness and senses were not orientated toward the illusion. Your future happiness offers the same illusion.

Secondly, you are turning your attention away from what really matters and that is contained within you. This would be akin to bandaging your ankle in the hope that your headache might go away. When you divert your attention from what is real within you, you acknowledge the pain and suffering by saying, *I see you and know that you are in pain.* Yet you do not allow a story to emerge from this witnessing.

To *Navigate Life* successfully and not get stuck into a *Parked* state, you need to be mindful of any part of you that causes you suffering. You see, the suffering itself is not about the story of pain. Rather, it is an invitation and an awakening to return back to wholeness. This is your default state and yet, you are likely to have assumed and picked up stories about yourself. These stories have come from outside influence, in order to create a mirage of who you think you need to be. Subsequently, when you are out of alignment with this wholeness, your ego automatically kicks in, in order to substantiate and validate this state. This is much like the bully who stands up at school defending his right to be a bully. Your ego assumes control in much the same manner.

Forgiving and healing the past should be approached with no other motive than unconditional healing. Many times people approach the healing process with the intention of unburdening themselves of past trauma in the hope that they will begin to feel good about themselves. Alternatively, they may also feel that forgiving and healing the past means wiping a clean slate and that all their troubles and concerns will melt away. This is obviously not the case and if you approach your healing from this perspective you will certainly be discouraged from continuing the healing process as other parts emerge.

Similarly, forgiving and healing the past does not mean forgetting what happened to you, since in doing so means denying that the past actually happened. Healing is a process which involves bringing peace and love within the present moment to any thoughts, beliefs or emotion that keeps you trapped in the past. You are trapped since you are not fully engaging in life.

Your repressed and toxic emotions also take up valuable energy since many of these emotions remain trapped within your muscular system and organs. Bringing the past into the present moment means bringing past memories and emotional trauma and igniting them within the present physical body. Dr John Sarno, who we spoke about in the previous chapters, showed that the emotions of anger and anxiety had the potential to create back pain within the clients that he saw. As he approached the healing process from a non-physical perspective, the client was able to heal by making peace with these toxic and destructive emotions that were taking up valuable resources within the physical body.

Another well recognized physician working in this area is Dr. Don Colbert who wrote the book *Deadly Emotions*. Dr. Colbert takes us through the various deadly emotions as seen from a physician's point of view and how they cause physiological destruction on the human body. He invites the reader to understand the deeper meaning behind the emotion and how to release and heal these toxic emotional states.

So let us revisit the forgiveness and healing process.

Firstly, awareness is the key to forgiving and healing the past. This may mean that although you do not have an accurate picture of the root cause of your problem, you are nonetheless aware that you carry unresolved aspects within. The process of awareness simply means becoming conscious of any aspect that causes you suffering.

The second component toward forgiveness involves self-examination. Recalling the work we covered in previous chapters on self-examination, this part involves the investigation with a compassionate heart toward the root cause of your suffering. Alternatively, if you feel that this process is far too arduous to undertake on your own, working alongside an understanding therapist will help you to heal and let go of past judgments.

The truth is that all you ever have is what is contained within this moment, but for now I want you to understand that your past does not equal your future. Your thinking and belief that it does, is what creates separation and suffering. Our minds are adept at predicting the future, since it is part of its makeup to perform that task. Yet sometimes, it overdoes its job by predicting circumstances that have no correlation to the present moment and future. Your only place of solitude is contained within the present moment, that is, when you are alive and awake to it. By awake, I mean without distractions, motives, beliefs or anything that threatens the pure joy and bliss of experiencing each moment as it is.

You do not see the world as it is. You see it as you are. Maybe you have heard this saying. What this means is that our worlds are shaped by our own unique perspectives, which is what makes the world such a diverse place. Each and every person on earth has their own filter through which they view life. Their perspectives may be shaped by beliefs from religion, sex, love, politics, environment and other so forth. What makes it interesting is that our past experiences of life, dictates how we perceive the present moment and the future. Our past may include our beliefs, thoughts, ideas and emotional constitution toward the world. What you see is a product of your individual perspective—no one sees what you see, even if they had the chance to look at life precisely from the location you are standing. Their judgment and perception is shaped from a different set of experiences, so they would never see your exact perspective.

To create an authentic experience of the present moment withholding judgment, labels, or stories, you must strive to release your learned programs and prejudices toward life and allow life to really reveal itself. Sometimes though, this may mean that what we see does not fit the model of what we believe is right. For example, you might have been taught to follow a certain political party, since your family and grandparents also followed this political party. However, you meet a wonderful partner who has all the loving qualities you could ever wish for, but he or she believes in the opposite political system. A part of you may feel compelled to judge and label your partner as inaccurate and it stands to reason that your partner should also share the same view.

Ultimately, we do not really know another person until we stand in their shoes and live their life.

The point worth making here is that we all have our own set of beliefs and past experiences that shape and create our current circumstances. Sometimes though, our present moment experience may be rooted in suffering and eternal problems. These come as a result of our personal biased that we have brought in to this present moment.

Now while some people may view this as a negative experience, I would suggest that it may be a positive experience insofar as the present moment serves as a measure of how much your past conditioning interferes with the pure awareness of this present moment. To create a more authentic experience in life, you must look at reviewing and examining your conditioned beliefs and perceptions by adjusting them to suit the present moment.

Taking the earlier example of opposing political views, it might mean approaching the topic with an openness to learn the other person's reasons for having these views, irrespective of whether you think they are wrong. Often in life we have adopted a set of beliefs and opinions that are deeply rooted and held with such conviction that we fail to recognize and authenticate the purity that each moment offers. By suspending our judgments about life, we approach every situation with an open heart and open mind, thus allowing multiple probabilities to simultaneously exist. This in essence is the beauty and simplicity of life when we abandon our notion of how life should *actually* be, and instead come from a place of pure awareness and allowing.

It takes a great deal of courage to face up to one's truth irrespective of whether they believe that truth to be false or inaccurate. I believe that our life takes on more meaning when we begin to examine any disowned aspects of ourselves which we have neglected, either intentionally or unintentionally. I like to look at life from the perspective of having acquired a level of understanding, given one's level of consciousness at the time. As you grow mentally, emotionally and spiritually, your filters also expand to allow you to see a world in a different way.

Judging yourself and others is too easy, since it shifts the blame from looking within and dealing with those parts we dislike. Those who remain *Parked* in life feel the need to label and judge others, believing that the world is wrong and they are right, when in fact what they are actually saying is**, I fail to recognize the part of me I have abandoned and so I choose to criticize and label you instead. I dislike that part of me, which I would rather not face**.

You can clearly see from this way of thinking that this person is playing the victim role by not recognizing that a part of them wishes to heal and express their authentic self.

Chapter Summary:

- Make it a priority to let go of things which you have found hard to forgive.

- Forgiving and healing the past means to recognize all that took place is a figment of your imagination.

- When you bring memories out of the past into the present moment, you are not awake and receptive to the NOW. You are drawing on memories and reliving painful experiences.

- You bring peace to the present moment when you release past hurt and transgression.

- Not forgiving the past means bringing the hurt into the present moment – it is like carrying a thorn in your sneakers.

- Make peace with the past through acceptance, with no other motive than to heal. You are not forgetting the past, just bringing peace to what happened.

- Painful memories are also stored in your physical body and organs.

- Go into silence and notice the parts of you that struggle to forgive.

- Bringing the past into your present, clouds your perception of experiencing the present moment.

- When you bring memories out of the past into the present moment, you are not awake or receptive to the pureness of the present moment.

- Victims never heal. They merely stroll through life with a wounded badge, carrying it like a trophy. They attack and blame others by shifting the focus of their unrecognized pain and suffering to someone else.

CHAPTER FIFTEEN
Navigate Your Emotional Well-being

Life Happens In The Present Moment

"The time is now, the place is here. Stay in the present. You can do nothing to change the past, and the future will never come exactly as you plan or hope for."

Dan Millman

To be more conscious and live a more conscious life means to be aware of yourself at each moment. If you are conscious, you are aware of the present moment and the fact that your inner self is awakened. It is being mindful and feeling the air entering and exiting your lungs. It is being present with your thoughts and emotions.

For example, have you ever gone on holiday and suddenly your perception of everything seems greater? You smell the fresh air, smile at the lush green trees and gorgeous flowers, and hear birds singing sweetly. You feel more alive and oftentimes happier because you have forgotten about the hundreds of thoughts running around in your mind. You are simply conscious of the beauty of your present surroundings. Those same beautiful surroundings could be in your neighborhood back home, but you are too focused on other things to notice. You do not take time to smell your own roses.

The deepest part of who we are, our consciousness or spirit, longs to be experienced. The problem is that it gets covered up by so many layers of negative things over the years. Childhood wounds, negative feelings, limiting beliefs, etc. pile on year after year and it gets harder and harder to connect with our spirit. To become more conscious requires a peeling away of these layer, one by one. The best way to do this is to become mindful of the present moment.

To live a more conscious life will require you to slow down, get quiet, and allow the painful wounds of the past to surface so you can process them and let them go, thus, digging down through layers to become more in tune with your spirit. As you do this, wounds begin to heal and wholeness arises. It is a beautiful transformation.

You might be thinking, who wants to go back to childhood and face old wounds? I understand, but it is an important process if you want to begin living a more conscious life.

Ponder these questions:

Are you happy with your life?
Do you love who you are?
Are you full of shame or pain?
Do you know your primary purpose in life?
Are your relationships up to par?

This is a great exercise that helps us reconnect in the present moment, rather than having our thoughts in the past or anticipating some future event. As an example, when was the last time you truly noticed the waves crashing into the shoreline and engaged your vision and hearing to absorb this?

Too often we take for granted that these things exist and blindly turn our attention and awareness away from the simple things in life, like the sound of birds on a spring morning. Such moments define the virtue of living a rich and fulfilling life. This is because we are aware and awake to the present moment in a state of gratitude.

So as you continue to spend time in Mother Nature, turn off your internal chatter and take the time to witness and observe your surroundings without the running commentary. Just as you used the earlier example of closing your eyes to envisage a particular scenario, you will have noticed at the time that your mind is less inclined to offer a dialogue during this process.

The purpose of these exercises is to reorient you toward the present moment, by canceling out your thoughts of the past or the future.

The wholeness that you feel when in the present moment is the same feeling that creative people and musicians feel when they are absorbed with their creative expression. They are filled with the beauty and rapture of life expressing itself through them. You have access to the same ability to stay grounded and present within the moment by bringing your awareness and attention back into the now.

Meditation is one form of practice that is effective in helping you maintain a present moment orientation. The practice of sitting alone in silence with your thoughts and observing your body, allows you to remain grounded within the present moment. You have probably heard the saying, *your body is in the present moment so why aren't your thoughts?* This simple yet powerful question reminds us to connect with our mind and body within the present moment.

So what can you do to remain in the present moment and be more conscious of doing so? Well for starters as you notice your thoughts drifting into the past or the future, gently nudge yourself back into the present moment by looking around to your immediate surroundings and becoming conscious and aware of these things.

As you observe your immediate surroundings you may begin to notice things which you previously had not drawn into your focus. It might be the design of your computer monitor, the texture of the seats you are sitting on or the way in which the indoor plant next to you shows off its green foliage, which is unusual in appearance.

Your brain is attempting to use historical information from your past in order to bring some sense of familiarity to the present moment, yet at the same time everything is fresh and alive. I urge you to view life with the same freshness and enthusiasm as that of a young child witnessing something new for the first time.

Another way to stay in the present moment is to pursue a passion, hobby or interest which engages all your senses. You may or may not already pursue this, yet if you do not I would encourage you to find something in your life that you are passionate toward and make more time for it in your life. You have probably read biographies on artists and musicians, describing the creative process of writing songs or playing music or creating masterful art pieces, as being a euphoric experience. They are lost and so absorbed with the creative process that time stands still and seems to pass in haste. I mentioned in an earlier chapter that when I am on stage speaking about my passion, I am so absorbed in the process that many times I actually forget what I said as soon as I step off stage.

In his book *The Time Paradox*, author Philip Zimbardo cites six different time perspectives, two of which are past, two present and two future orientated. They are:

- Past negative
- Past positive
- Present fatalistic
- Present hedonistic
- Future
- Transcendental future

We are orientated toward living these six perspectives that tend to shape and influence the way we view reality. You have probably heard about the study in which a famous classical violinist was playing his violin, a Stradivarius, in a busy New York subway. (If you are not aware of this type of violin, they were constructed during the 1700s, which was known as Stradivarius golden period, which sold for \$16 000 000 at an auction.)

What was interesting to note here was due to their thoughts being on the future, many of these commuters failed to recognize and acknowledge a world renowned musician playing this exquisite instrument. This observation shows that when people live with the future as their orientation, they tend to neglect the present moment since they are consumed mentally about the future. I mention this since I am sure you have been responsible for living in the future in your mind at the mercy of missing out on the beauty of the present moment.

Those who are future orientated may be prone to anxiety and worry since their mind is repeatedly focused on a scenario playing out in a certain way. *You can do nothing to change the past, and the future will never come exactly as you plan or hope for.* This thought reminds us that the future never arrives as we expect or hope for and subsequently we miss out on the present moment because our minds are fast forward into the future while the present moment is taking shape.

So **how do we orientate ourselves toward living in the present moment when much of our lives is ruled by the future?** We plan so many of our future events, such as birthdays, meetings, holidays etc. Whilst it is okay to make future plans, doing so repeatedly at the risk of missing out on the present moment removes us from the real beauty and fulfillment of life since all we are doing is living in an anticipated future event while the present moment is the reality that we actually have.

My suggestion is to come from a place of acceptance. Accept anything that shows up in your current reality, rather than trying to escape it in your mind. Acceptance does not mean apathy, it means embracing the present moment for what it offers and then aligning your thoughts and emotions to creating a new future.

For example, you might be dissatisfied in your current career and find your day-to-day work mentally and emotionally exhausting. Rather than focusing on the negative aspects toward future events, such as the time you finish work, the weekend or even a holiday. It might be in your best interest to accept that this moment is what it is and create new and empowering thoughts that align with how you wish to create a more empowered future.

When you are caught up in a pursuits or moment that is enriched with joy and satisfaction, you wish for more of the same energy to unfold.

In the final part of the book I will outline a number of valuable lessons that will help guide you toward *Navigating Life*. It is essential that you put them to practice in your daily life but more on that later.

Chapter Summary:

- Be in nature more often and notice things—learn to observe. Do not let your mind make commentary.

- When your thoughts stray into the past or future, reconnect with the present moment.

- Pursue your passion, music, art etc, which allows you to stay present.

- Develop mindfulness to keep you present and grounded in the moment.

- Do not get caught up in the future since it never arrives and creates more misery and suffering when life does not go as planned.

- Approach life from a perspective of total acceptance without an agenda other than to show up and be here and now.

- The book, *The Time Paradox*, talks about different perceptions of time: past, present and future orientated.

CHAPTER SIXTEEN

Living the Lessons

Harness Your Potential

> *"Follow your bliss and the universe will open doors for you where there were once only walls."*

Joseph Campbell

In the previous chapters we discussed a blueprint for *Navigating Life* by focusing on eight areas of your life in which to draw your focus. As you attend to these eight blueprints, by making them a part of your life, you will see and reap the benefits that these valuable lessons offer you in time. I have discovered both personally and on a professional level that as we attend to these eight areas, wonderful and amazing events and circumstances take hold in our lives. We become more than we are because we begin to accept more of ourselves. We reach for a greater and higher potential as we will work towards our highest version of ourselves.

In this section I will provide you with six lessons that are fundamental in helping you take charge and *Navigate* your life successfully. As we move through the coming chapters, you should by now already have a firm understanding of whether you are *Navigating Life*, *Parked* or somewhere in between. At the end of these chapters you will find a detailed questionnaire that will help you gain an insight as to where you sit on the continuum. I suggest that you review this questionnaire from time to time as a means of gauging whether you remain *Parked* and stagnant, or indeed if you are successfully *Navigating Life*.

Do not view anything in your life as negative or untoward. View it as a platform in which to grow and move toward that which you desire. So how does one harness their potential and why is it important to *Navigating Life*? Harnessing your potential means to take ownership of your innate talents, skills and creativity in order to become the best version of yourself. We were all born with amazing potential which lays dormant until we choose to access it. Some of us have to work harder than others in order to reveal that potential. It may come early in life or in some cases later in life. Your concern should not be when success is bestowed upon you, but rather to work towards excellence.

The most successful and talented people who have achieved international recognition within their area of expertise have pursued that which they are passionate about and makes their heart sing. They will tell you that had they earned no money they still would have pursued their vocation, because it brought them great joy. When discussing these people earlier we saw that they continually connect with their mind and body to reveal the best version of themselves. They harness their true potential by seeking to build on what they know and understand. They expand their awareness and consciousness and have a childlike curiosity about the world. They are genuinely interested in the joy that their pursuit brings them, and being aware of this allows them to bring the same level of joy and passion to others in the world. We can say that since they are connecting with their hearts, and the heart is where love resides, they are sharing love with humanity. Love is one of the highest sources of energy in the world and according to Dr. David Hawkins' *Map of Consciousness*, it calibrates at one of the highest levels on the logarithmic scale. When you connect from a deeper place filled with love, you invite higher frequencies of energy to permeate through your mind and body. You begin to work with this high frequency which vibrates at such a powerful intensity that it feeds the hearts and minds of those you connect with.

Remember Joseph Campbell said, *the universe will open doors for you where there were once only walls.* He invites us to connect with our hearts and minds by pursuing that which gives us joy and in turn we begin to share that passion and joy with others. It similarly connects and reaches within our heart and mind. So harnessing your potential means connecting with the higher source of energy based in love and sharing that love with others in the pursuit of service.

When you frame it from this perspective, you begin to see that what you do on a smaller scale has the potential to impact and touch the lives of many people because you are connecting with a source of energy that is available to us all.

When you understand that life conspires in your favor, you will see that it is how you think about situations that may seem untoward and are in fact working in your favor. You see, most of the time we do not have a clear picture of how our life is unfolding because we are so caught up in the drama of our lives that we fail to see that each aspect of the drama connects to form the greater picture of your evolution.

Go out and greet life with the passion and enthusiasm that resides within you. Do not wait for life to happen to you because surely you will be dissatisfied with what shows up since it will not be according to your desires. Many people give up on life far too quickly because they fail to see results in the initial stages. The way I see it, giving up is way too easy and does not build character and personal growth.

So allow life to flow through you because you are life and the expression of life. Your desires and your wants have been bestowed upon you by a benevolent universe that dearly wants you to succeed and excel. This benevolent universe is not so thoughtless as to hand you your desires without building strength of character and resolve and so it masterfully orchestrates roadblocks and setbacks, asking of you to overcome these, so that as you draw near to the prize, you will become a better version of yourself—one worthy of claiming the prize.

Greet life with enthusiasm and passion, for if you knew how valuable your gifts and talents are then you would not rest one minute in sharing these with the world. Now this does not mean that you will only experience joy and happiness throughout your life, and it would be remiss of me to suggest this Pollyanna type existence. What I am offering is a deeper sense of fulfillment that is steeped in a passion and desire that overwhelms all the tough and bad moments of your life. It is like the Olympic athlete who strives to represent his or her country in the Olympics. Given the Olympics come around every four years, undoubtedly within that period the athlete trains and gathers their physical resources in order to show up at the Olympics in the best form they can. They never anticipate that injury and setbacks will occur along the way and yet these setbacks can derail the athlete by thwarting their enthusiasm toward training.

The athlete has such an undeniable commitment, and resolve to succeed that they are willing to overcome any hurdle or obstacle that they face. This could include injuries. They are at war with themselves mentally, emotionally and physically as they strive to reveal the best version of themselves and showcase this to millions of people around the world.

I suggest you to adopt a similar way of life by working toward a better version of yourself. View your day to day work as your training, much like the athletes train. Show up to life with the best version of yourself knowing well that each thought, belief and emotion that you entertain, draws you closer toward the person you wish to be.

You can achieve anything that you set your mind to as long as you have a deep conviction without contemplating failure.

Undoubtedly, if and when setbacks present themselves, your deepest conviction is so strong and powerful that it has the potential to dominate and override the lower states of doubt and fear. Insist that you will succeed, even if you do not know how. Just believe with your entire mind and body that you have what it takes to harness your potential.

We are advised that if you work hard enough, success will undoubtedly be there to greet you. I am not sure where this model came from and I would suggest that it is possibly fraught with danger, since it implies a cause and effect model for success. Rather than pursue success, which in my opinion will elude you, pursue excellence in your area of expertise. When you pursue excellence instead of success, you are pursuing the higher state of success because inevitably what you do will be borne out of passion and love and will be represented in your work; therefore success becomes imminent as a by-product of pursuing excellence.

You see the many great leaders, and those who have achieved world-class success, have done so because they started small. They chose to pursue their passion and interest on a smaller scale, perhaps not even considering that it would amount to anything greater than self-interest born through passion. Inevitably as they pursued their interests with passion and enthusiasm this became evident to others along the way until they stepped into their moment of success through hard work, persistence and determination.

What if you have been led to believe that pursuing your passion is a false ideal? Whatever others have told you about pursuing your passion is also an incorrect assumption based on the life path that they have chosen. People often advise you that you cannot achieve what you set out to do because it is fraught with the unknown, which may involve risk and financial setbacks. I suggest that you resist the temptation to listen to such advice.

Many comedians started out telling jokes to their families when they were young and I would dare say they were ridiculed by loved ones for even suggesting that they could be successful as a comedian. Despite this they pursued their passion by harnessing their potential, which inevitably paid off if they stuck at it long enough.

To harness your potential is to successfully *Navigate Life* because you are pursuing that which you love. When you are pursuing that which you love, whilst sharing it with others, you stand in the place that the universe has orchestrated for you. You are listening to the silent whisper of the heart, which we describe in earlier chapters as speaking with a silent and intuitive whisper. Go there often to connect and discover the silent voice within you, which is calling you back to reconnect with your authentic self.

I do not know about you, but when I die I want to have used every morsel of talent, genius and skill I have. And to be the best that I can be, by being of service to others while sharing my passion, enthusiasm and joy with the world. Mitch Albom wrote a fabulous book about this very essence called *Tuesdays with Morrie*, in which the author reconnects with his college professor and mentor in the last few months of his life. Morrie recounts the innumerable lessons that he gained throughout his life, and shares them with Mitch. The dying professor sums up his life's lessons, themed around the concepts of love, acceptance, communication, openness and happiness.

How do you wish to leave your mark on the world? If you work backwards from this realization, you can see that everything that you do from this point in time will be cast upon you during your final hours on this earth. Now is the time to make it count by being the best that you can be. Refuse to play small because playing small is way too easy and comfortable and brings with it little or no rewards. Your successes awaits you on the other side of your comfort zone and in order to get there, you must painstakingly work through and collapse any obstacle, whether it be mental, emotional or physical, in order to create the life that you wish to live.

You know no one will really care if you pursue your passion or not other than yourself. Sure your friends, family and loved ones may express dissatisfaction that you have to give it your best, but ultimately who really cares in the end? During your final hours those people will not be around to summarize how you missed the valuable opportunities that were made favorable to you because you were too afraid to harness your potential. People and circumstances come and go from your life as quickly as the breath that you inhale. The world around you will continue, irrespective of whether you stepped up and take on the chance to become your best.

Ultimately, what really matters is the connection you have with yourself. What matters is that you have listened to the calling of your heart inviting you to pursue and become all that you can be.

What matters is that you took the chance and the risk to live to your potential by harnessing every talent, skill and effort to follow your hearts calling. Determination and persistence is something that cannot be taught to others. Certainly we can read about it and understand it at an intellectual level, yet until we embody these two qualities and understand it at a cellular level, will we not know what it means to have harnessed our potential.

Chapter Summary:

- Step into your life and claim it. Find out what makes your heart sing and pursue it with passion.

- Live with all your senses. Do not wait to allow life to happen to you.

- Go out and greet it with enthusiasm. Become the best version of yourself you can be. You can make it happen if you try and never give up.

- Pursue that which you love and are passionate about – strive for excellence and not success.

- Think excellence in all you do – even if you sweep floors, for it is not in the doing, but the enthusiasm and passion you bring to your job that will be noticed.

- I want to retire from this life completely wrung out like a damp cloth, like every cell of my mind and body has been used to provide value and service to others. What is your wish at the final hour?

- Determination and consistency will always win. Develop an inner resolve that no-one can diminish.

CHAPTER SEVENTEEN

Living the Lessons

Choosing Navigate Life When Parked

"It is better to live your own destiny imperfectly than to live an imitation of somebody else's life with perfection."

Anonymous, The Bhagavad Gita

In the previous chapter I invited you to harness your potential as one of the lessons for *Navigating Life*. We looked at ways in which you can take advantage of your potential by stepping into your power and harnessing your potential through your gifts, your talents and skills. In this chapter we will look at ways to move from a *Parked* state to *Navigating* state.

In one of the earlier chapters of the book we defined the two areas by looking at what it means to be *Parked* versus *Navigating life*.

We also saw the life's roadmap which depicted the two various states of *Parked* and *Navigating* represented by two circles with a transition period in between. The purpose of the roadmap was to represent the various stages in cycles that one typically undergoes in the eight aspects shown in the *Navigating Life* wheel.

What is worth appreciating from the life roadmap diagram is the various movement and energy on both sides. Whilst the *Parked* state may be stagnant there is still a cycle within it that is depicted by the preparation and recovery phases. The transitional period shown in grey, represents the crossover from the two dimensions as the various interplay between the two. The *Navigating* phase on the right-hand side also has two aspects to it that are depicted by the ascension and the completion phase. Both these two areas represent the highest point or pinnacle in one's movements or evolution and subsequently the transition of that energy to either higher or lower states.

On the left-hand side of the diagram I have purposely created dotted lines in red to represent the recurring aspect of the *Parked* state. These dotted lines are knots represented in the *Navigating* phase, since we tend to stay stuck or *Parked* more often than we are *Navigating Life*. It is positively assumed that if you are in a *Navigating* state, then you are achieving a level of success within your life.

It is important to recognize when you are *Parked* and to take action by moving from this stagnant state to a higher energy, such as *Navigating Life.*

Your life is an organic and harmonious flow of energy, which is moving from either a *Parked* to a *Navigating* state or vice versa. Your reality is giving you feedback via your thoughts, emotions and external occurrences as to which energy source you are predominantly working with. It is worth re-emphasizing that there are no mistakes in life, only the opportunity to self-correct by appreciating the feedback that life offers and by responding to it.

The single biggest resource that you have available to you at all times is the ownership of your thoughts.

By tending to your thoughts in order to create a new destiny template, it is imperative that you become mindful of your thoughts as we suggested previously. This has the net effect of drawing them to your awareness, which then takes note of these limiting or destructive thought patterns if and when they emerge. We also examined the basis of the thoughts as having little value until you attach yourself to these thoughts and give meaning to them. I suggested that you do not create a story around these thoughts by giving them more energy than they deserve.

If you review the work in the earlier chapters in the Blueprint for the *Navigating Life* section, you will note that we spent some time understanding the nature of thoughts and how they drive and influence our emotional state. Often people encounter untoward situations in their life and feel compelled to rectify these by tending to them whilst unduly neglecting their inner world.

Your problems are never "out there," for you must go within in order to reclaim the power that is forever available to you. It is been passed down through the ages that our external world starts at the level of the mind. The following saying, *as within, so without,* is testament to much of what I have been conveying to you. **Focus and tend to your inner being by being aware of your nature and tending to your inner landscape as the need arises**.

This is the whole basis to *Navigating Life*, and your journey to freedom is the understanding that life is perpetual, cyclical and creative in nature. There are ebbs and flows and movement of energy that predicts and controls circumstances in your life once you adhere and learn to work with these forces. Learning to work with these forces does not mean to succumb to life and become a victim to your circumstances, rather that you understand that there are indeed powerful universal laws and truths that we must learn to abide by and work with.

Working with this energy means that you are in a powerful position to not remain stuck and stagnant in any area of your life. Rather than becoming a victim to life's circumstances and feeling that you have been hard done by, *Navigating Life* empowers you to understand and appreciate that there are equal and opposite forces coexisting at the same time and that neither of these forces and energy are good or bad. Once you aligned yourself with the truth of your deepest self, you are in a powerful position to be a conscious creator because you are empowered to take action on your thoughts, which resonate with the deepest part of you.

Life is advising you to pick and choose those areas of your life that bring you the greatest joy and satisfaction and allow the lower energies to naturally fall away. Recall in the previous chapters on the blueprint for life, we spoke about letting go of things that do not serve you. These things which do not serve you included people, places, circumstances and events that do not resonate with your deepest self. I think we overcomplicate things by becoming too attached to these aspects of our lives as our ego feels insignificant when we're unable to control and manage certain parts of our lives effectively.

Whilst to the novice mind, this may seem as a failure as things begin to collapse and fall away, to the trained mind this is in fact a blessing in disguise as life is advising you of the areas that you need to pay greater attention to. So circumstances in your life may initially appear as catastrophic, are in fact life working itself out for your greater benefit. In such times suspend your judgment of anything that appears on the surface to be a negative experience until you have a clearer picture of what is taking place. For this reason there are no accidents and no negative experiences in life unless we decide to assign meaning to these occurrences.

As we referred to in earlier chapters relating to the life's view diagram, that even being stuck is an opportunity to move forward since life reflects back to you a sense of disengagement, offering you the opportunity to take action. If you fail to take action then you may fall into a rut and continue the repetitive *Parked* cycle.

You are a conscious creator, creating your version of events and circumstances at a micro level. Your universe co-creates these circumstances of your life in joyful harmony when you connect and align with the deepest aspect of your inner being. This deepest self is the expression of life and holds all the answers to your questions. Therefore, you cannot make any mistakes once you are in perfect harmony and synchronized with the universal energy of life.

Whilst I appreciate that we are merely a minute component of a greater force that is active in the universe, we still have the ability to consciously create the circumstances of our life by being in alignment and in harmony with our deepest self.

You have the power to change your thoughts, your words and your actions within each moment. What you think today creates your tomorrow. So the power of thought is one of the most powerful tools available to man and it is worth your time in understanding and befriending your thoughts. Rather than have them overwhelm you with the incessant internal chatter that plays in your mind.

You may have noticed there is a time lag between your desires and the fulfillment of these desires. This is both a positive and negative situation in that it allows you to be aware of your predominant thought landscape and make any adjustments in order to create more self-empowering thoughts.

It may seem to be a passive experience waiting for what you desire to come to fruition as it may take longer than you wish. The purpose of this is to allow you time to appreciate and come to terms with that which you desire. By doing so, you send a message to the universe that you are absolutely positive that your desires are in alignment with your deepest self and wish these to be realized. The time lag allows you to identify in that period any other adjustments you want before your desires manifest.

Therefore, your thoughts are both perpetual and creative in nature because they turn into things. Once these things appear in your reality it is often too late to send them back or change your mind. You need to be sure of what you want before creating it by aligning yourself with your inner world. As previously stated, as within so without, serves as both an affirmation and a reminder that what we think about, eventually makes its way into our reality whether we like it or not.

As mentioned earlier on in the book, change from *Parked* to *Navigate* can take time and be difficult, therefore, I urge you to do your own research on the change model and pay particular attention to the six phases of change. Knowing these phases occur allows us to take the foot off the accelerator and rest assured that most times everything is working itself out for our greater benefit. We simply need to remain calm, poised and at peace in the knowledge that we are changing our emotional, mental and physical landscape and in doing so the resistance that we offer is understandable and valid.

Chapter Summary:

- This chapter is about recognizing the ebb and flow of life and understanding that things do not remain the same forever. Your current reality is shaped as a result of the thoughts you previously held. Change your thoughts and change your destiny.

- Recognize that life is cyclical. Know when you are *Parked* and take action to keep the momentum moving in your favor.

- Do not remain stuck in a rut and let life happen to you. Be proactive and make conscious decisions on what you would like to manifest in your life.

- You have the power to change your thoughts, your words and your actions within each moment. What you think today creates your tomorrow.

- Change is hard at the best of times. It takes time and patience so does not feel compelled to change your life quickly.

- *Parked* and *Navigating* is simply the movement of energy from one state to another.

- Life is reflecting back your current mental and emotional position – take note and adjust your course.

CHAPTER EIGHTEEN
Living the Lessons

Problems are ALWAYS Opportunities

"Life is what happens to you when you are busy making other plans."

John Lennon

In part three of living the lessons, we will look at how problems can in fact give rise to opportunities instead of setting you back and causing stress and worry. Problems exist at the level of the mind, as that is the way our mind is conditioned. The result allows a problem to either overwhelm us, or in the case of successful people, become an opportunity to gain something. This may seem to be over optimistic, but I would suggest that the process of life is in fact opportunistic.

The universal energy of life is conspiring in your favor in order to bring you events and circumstances for your greatest good. It is just that we often get in the way of ourselves by limiting the level of fulfillment, abundance and prosperity that is readily available to us through disempowering thoughts and the accompanying emotions that go with them. So if there are problems in your life that are causing you concern or posing stress and worry, I invite you for a moment to see ways in which these problems may give way to possible solutions or even realize opportunities.

It is difficult for the rational mind to come up with answers, yet if you contemplate enough, there are favorable opportunities even in the direst situations. Your problems arise as a way of signaling to you that your thought landscape is out of balance. Remember that life is reflecting back to you what you think about. In order to change the circumstances of our lives, we must look to our thoughts as a valuable tool that creates our reality.

Favorable solutions must exist in order to complement the problem, since life is a reflection of dualities. This is evident when you are stressed and anxious, via the two branches of your nervous system, which serve to regulate your heart rate in such a state. Similarly at the same time, whilst your body is in a fight or flight response, your digestive system is inhibited in order to facilitate a much-needed blood supply to the peripheral organs. In this way nature has a plan that serves to preserve the body's systems without causing long term health concerns.

Life is what happens to you when you are busy making other plans, is a well-known song-line of John Lennon. **The creative force of the universe is forever working in your favor but only once you let go and trust in the process of life.** Once you are able to do this, the problems become solvable, because the mind that created the problem is also capable of finding a solution. It does not matter how long it takes to manifest the solution, but merely knowing that it exists, coupled with a belief is enough to create and invite the solution to make its way into your life.

Your life story is the product of the questions that you put out into the universe whether they are conscious or unconscious. You are living the answers to your questions, for the universe is forever answering your questions if you choose to listen or tune in to the correct frequency. In order to tune into the correct vibrational frequency of the creative intelligence, it is essential that you become the conduit for that energy to make its way into your space.

To do this, you must abandon all preconceived ideas, thoughts and perceptions on how solutions make their way into your life. You must surrender your attachment to the timing of how these solutions are received for even that can derail the receiving process. In order to start seeing the solutions to your problems you need to not only create the mental space for these solutions but to also create the emotional space from which possible solutions enter your heart space.

We discovered that the creative intelligence of the universe is vested in love. Therefore, all probabilities of solutions exist on a level of consciousness, which vibrates on a frequency of love. What this means is that if your thoughts are out of alignment, and this relates to greed, anxiety, anger, jealousy or any other lower thought forms, then you are preventing a higher energetic frequency that is aligned with love to make its way into your life. My offering to you is to align with this vibrational frequency of love in order to receive the best possible solution to your problems.

One of my favorite sayings when I am in the midst of a problem is, *how would love respond in this situation?* By viewing your problem from this higher perspective you invite a higher intelligence to find expression through the best possible scenario. Let me reiterate that your logical mind cannot possibly create the perfect solution to your problems better than what the universal mind can. So in order to transcend your problem, invite this higher mind to create the best possible solution, without forming attachments to how and when it makes its way into your life. Your job is to be open to receive and accept what shows up by disabling your preconditioned and preconceived ideas of what is deemed an effective solution.

The more you operate from this level of awareness and consciousness, the more solutions you will invite into your life with the least resistance. All the answers to all problems exist on a level of awareness in space time. All we have to do is dial into the frequency and be in a receptive state to receive the answers without casting judgments on how and when our problems will be answered.

Often, we assume that our problems occur to hinder our progress or that the universal life force is conspiring against us. The truth remains that any untoward circumstances or events occurring in our lives has been called for in order to help and guide us along our paths. An example, if you wish to be a successful writer, then life will test you by presenting you with circumstances and events that will test your resolve to see how much you really want to achieve your goal. Furthermore, in order to become a successful writer you must have the inner determination, patience and courage in order to pursue that desire. What better way to test this inner resolve by presenting you with situations which allow inner growth?

You could say the same scenario exists in all of life, particularly in the animal kingdom. If we look to young animals, such as tigers or lions, you will have noticed that in order for the cubs to grow into mature hunters and predators, they must face every obstacle and challenge from an early age. Mother Nature does not intend to overpower the young cubs, but it does present situations and circumstances that enable the cubs to learn to fend for themselves as inevitably they will need these skills and knowledge in order to sustain life as mature adults.

Whilst I acknowledge that this is an oversimplified view of Mother Nature, it nonetheless represents a concept in which we can adapt and apply to our own lives.

Another example; Imagine for a moment that you are looking for a new job, after having recently finished working in a job that did not provide you with the creative space you required to prosper or show your talents. So whilst sending out job applications and resumes, there is the likelihood that out of five applications, you might get knocked back four times. Now on the surface receiving four rejection letters can be daunting and self-defeating in some ways. But what if I were to advise you that it will take another fifteen job applications in which you will receive a further twelve rejection letters in order to arrive at the best job offer. Would you still proceed knowing this?

The point is that we do not have that information available to us. On the surface, rejection and failure can be disheartening at the best of times, especially when we are eager and wish to get ahead in life. But you see the prize inevitably exists at the end of your search, it just took fifteen attempts and twelve rejections in order to find a job that is to your liking.

Successful people have learnt not to think in terms of good or bad situations, rather they suspend judgment of the events and circumstances until they have a full and complete picture of what is taking place. Successful people, like all other people are subject to the same failures and setbacks as everyone else, it is just that they do not interpret the failures and setbacks as a dead end or give up. They learn to harness the tools and resources from the experience in the journey that becomes a valuable aid to help them create the future possibilities.

Try to foster the same level of thinking by expecting situations to unfold in your favor by developing a strong and powerful belief and conviction. This inner conviction is not concerned with the logistics, instead it requires fostering a deep inner knowing and belief that everything is developing and unfolding exactly as it should, even when things appear catastrophic on the surface.

Your single greatest success in life will come from your inner belief that advises you to continue on life's path irrespective of how many setbacks and failures you encounter.

The *Navigating* person looks at life with optimism and enthusiasm, and finds evidence of this when it appears. However, the *Parked* individual focuses on the negativity in their life and life will always prove them right. Auto inventor Henry Ford said, *whether you think you can, or you think you can't—you are right.* The truth of this statement exemplifies the essence that life supports you until you learn to correctly align your thoughts with your deepest desires. Life waits for you to take the first step, but irrespective of whether that step is a positive or a negative one, will determine what shows up in your life.

It has taken some of the greatest and most successful people on earth an entire lifetime to form themselves into the people that they have become. Whilst we would like to think and acknowledge that success can be attained far more easily than this, the consequence is that anything that is easily attained may be easily lost.

Chapter Summary:

- Problems exist at the level of the mind; we must reorientate ourselves to possible solutions by asking quality questions.

- When you orientate your senses toward the possibility that there exist things that are beyond your understanding, you awaken to the infinite possibilities that life can yield.

- The life you live is a product of the questions you send forth into the universe. You are living your questions.

- Before assuming anything as bad, give it some time and ask yourself, *what could be possibly going on behind the scene to yield a positive outcome?*

- Problems exist to facilitate your inner growth; your inner growth allows you to deal with life's situations more harmoniously and favorably.

- Successful people do not think in terms of good or bad, they think in terms of OPPORTUNITIES. By thinking this way, you orientate your mind toward solutions.

- Everything you experience "out there" is reflecting back your inner landscape. If you do not like what is out there, readjust your inner world to coincide with what you would like to see.

CHAPTER NINETEEN
Living the Lessons

Give Meaning to Your Life

*"Life has no meaning. Each of us has meaning and we bring it to life.
It is a waste to be asking the question when you are the answer."*

Joseph Campbell

In the previous chapter we discussed the concept that all problems are
a gateway toward possibility and thus opportunities if we orientate our
mind toward finding the gift contained within each life experience.
In this chapter we will add to this concept by helping you formulate
questions that will empower you to find meaning in any of life situations.

Earlier in the book I quoted Shakespeare, who said *there* is *nothing either
good or bad but thinking make it so.* Therefore, if we continue along this
line of thought we can conclude that every experience in life presents
us with an opportunity for inner growth at some level. What precludes
the gateway of opportunity unfolding is the quality of the questions that
one asks.

For example, if you are in a hurry to get to work for an appointment
and in doing so you receive a speeding fine, then a person who is not
orientated toward looking for the gift of the experience will view it
as something bad happening to them and laments about the cost of
speeding fines and how unfairly they were treated. To the opportunistic
mind, this person will look for the gift of the experience by seeing it as

an opportunity to slow down and be present and grounded and that the universe is throwing them a life-line, rather than risk being involved in a car accident. At this point the consequences may be far direr than a brief monetary hit to the pocket.

As you *Navigate Life* you too are following the same route via the level of questions that you are directing to the Universe. The Universe, much like a shop retailer is constantly responding to your requests irrespective of whether you deem the situation to be positive or negative. It is important that you examine the quality of questions that you pose, whether they are conscious or unconscious. Now while this requires some introspective consideration, taking the time to examine one's predominant thought process has the potential to shape your future in a positive way.

Are your questions coming from a place of lack or resistance? Do you feel like a victim in the process of life? Do you compare yourself to those who are doing it better or more successful then you are, wishing that you have the same opportunities?

Well if you answered "yes" to any of these questions, chances are that the reason that you are feeling this way is largely attributed to the quality of the questions that you are entertaining.

So, how do we create a new script from our current level of awareness? The answer to this is simply by being more present in your current situation and asking positive questions that lead to successful outcomes. As we stated earlier, there is always a positive or negative lesson that is contained with each life experience. No two people can have the same experience and yield the same lesson, since their minds are vastly difference and will create two different conclusions as a result.

The quality of the questions that you pose will determine the quality of life that you set out to achieve. So how does one create value in their questions to create the quality of life which they seek? Remember that we live in a vibratory universe where every thought you have vibrates at a higher frequency, which is in accordance and vibrational harmony with a greater intelligence or vibrates at a lower frequency, which is in disharmony with the intelligence.

The mind is astute at finding evidence toward the contrary of that which you seek. Therefore, you must engage positive thoughts, matched with higher vibrational energy that is in alignment with your future desires.

To create your quality life, be willing to pose quality questions. *What are your current lessons? What is life teaching you? Is it in the form of an experience or to draw your awareness toward something? Are you seeking the answers to your questions or simply playing the victim role in the hope that your situation will change? It takes time, faith and patience to practice detachment and you will slip back into your old ways along the way.* In each situation you face in life, start small by releasing worries and anxieties about how your problems will turn out.

Ask yourself the following questions: *Who will I be when I achieve this quality of life? What will my life look like when I have achieved this quality of life?* By working backward from your empowering questions you will have gained a picture of how to live life from this present moment.

I am certain at some point you have imagined how your life might change if you acquired a certain object or achieved a certain milestone or goal. When you allow your imagination to take hold, by asking questions, you invite a higher mind to dream of possibilities to create that future. Focus on empowering questions that are positive in nature, framed around and affirming outcome. Earlier we spoke about negative questions empowering negative outcomes, so it holds true that orientating your senses toward that which you wish to see in your life will yield the greatest results.

Use the above suggested questions as a way to create the answers that you wish to live.

Living the Lessons

Many people believe that to give meaning to life requires a pilgrimage to a desolate part of the world, working with indigenous tribes and being of service. While I do not discount the value of this selfless work, the truth is that we can give meaning to our life through our own power to define what is important to us. You already have the power to create meaning and purpose in your life, not so much in what you do, but in what it means to you and the meaning you attach to it. For instance a person sweeping floors can define their life as being meaningful if the money they earn provides adequate food and shelter for their family. *What you do does not create the meaning—it is the meaning you assign to what you do that is important.* The meaning you hold toward something is represented from a deeper place within you. That is to say that the *act* or *thing* does not in itself define you.

For example, many people arrive at a crossroad in their life, which is generally around middle age where they feel they must achieve a certain status or have acquire a certain level of recognition. They cleverly recite their rewards and achievements believing all too well that having accomplished or acquired these things, that they will be more content and have achieved their purpose in life.

In truth, many of these same people feel a sense of lack and emptiness because the pursuit or goal was not imbued with passion and purpose. They failed to acknowledge the deeper meaning behind why they set out to achieve that goal in the first place. They lost their way in the pursuit of it. You have the power to create and define the meaning you attach to everything you do—including your life's purpose—by creating it yourself. It might contradict what society defines as successful but does it really matter?

Even defining success in itself is arbitrary and may be challenged in many ways. Success is not something you acquire as it remains elusive if you pursue it. Success is a state of being. You can be successful handing out mailbox letter drops if it brings you happiness and fulfillment. Society has attempted to place a square around what it values as a success and for this reason there are many wealthy, unhappy and unfulfilled people. These same people find joy and happiness when they lose themselves in service to others through volunteer work or any social community charitable work.

The key is to not allow yourself to be defined by what others view as success, since in doing so, you will be living up to an unattainable goal, one that you will never reach. Redefine success by giving it your definition as opposed to someone else's. The more we attempt to live by a set of rules and precepts, the more we are under the influence of other's ideals. It is essential that one defines their own level of success and not aim to achieve success but rather to become and embody success. *Have you ever noticed that successful people attract successful situations and events into their life? This is not because of who they are but because of who they are being.*

So to create meaning in one's life, it is important that you simplify your life by finding out what is important to you. I suggest that you make a list and take the time to contemplate what the most important aspects of your life are and eliminate anything which competes against the pursuit of this importance. For example, if you list health, family, relationships and career, then you have a strong representation of what brings you fulfillment, joy and happiness since these are the areas where you feel most appreciated and rewarded. It holds value that you would spend and allocate much of your resources and energy tending toward these aspects of your life and subsequently give less energy toward other areas of your life.

Simplify life by determining what is important to you. Old people will tell you that they wish they could have given more time and energy to those things that were important to them.

There is a classic story which embodies this principle.

There once was a professor of philosophy, who in front of his class, took a large empty pot of jam and without saying a word, began to fill it with golf balls.

Then he asked his students if the jar was full. The Students replied; YES.

The professor then took a box full of marbles and poured the marbles into the pot of jam. The marbles filled the gaps in between the Golf balls. The Professor asked the students again if the jar was full. Again, they replied: YES.

At that point, the professor took a bag of sand and poured it into the pot of jam. Of course, the sand filled all the remaining gaps. The professor asked again if the jar was full. The Students unanimously answered; YES.

The professor then added two cups of coffee to the contents of the jar, thus filling the small gaps between the grains of sand. The students started laughing. After they stopped, the professor said; "I want you to realize that the pot of jam represents Life.

The golf balls represent the very important things in Life, such as family, children, and health, everything you are passionate about. Our lives would still be full even if we'd lost everything else and these were the only things that remained.

The marbles are the other things that count in our lives such as work, house, car, etc ...

The sand represents everything else, all the small things in life.

If we had first poured sand into the jar, there would not have been any room left for the marbles or the golf balls.

It is the same thing in Life. If we put all our energy and all our time into the small things, we will never have any time/space left for the things that really matter.

Pay attention to the things that are really important to your happiness. Play with your children, take time to go to the doctor, have dinner with your spouse/partner, exercise or take time to enjoy your favorite pass-times.

There will always be time to do the cleaning and fix the taps on the kitchen sink.

Take care of the golf balls first, of the things that really matter. Choose your priorities, the rest is just sand."

One of the students then raised a hand and asked what the coffee meant.

The professor smiled and said: "It is good that you ask. I only added coffee to show that although your lives may seem full and busy, there is always room for a cup of coffee with a friend."

The point of the story as you no doubt understood is that many of life's events come and go, although the things that remain important to you should be acknowledged and revered since these are the things that really matter. Life can pass us all too quickly if we are not willing to embrace the experiences and remain grounded in the present moment, which is a true blessing. Do not allow yourself to reflect back on your past or hope for a better future since that takes away from the beauty that is the NOW. Prioritizing what is important to you and making that your focus allows you to simplify life and live it with passion, rather than trying to fill the jar with meaningless things that ultimately do not matter. When we re-engineer our lives from reverse, the premises is that we are looking at life from the perspective of being on our death bed and contemplating what is really important to us.

By determining what is important allows you to orientate your energy and resources toward those things by making space and room for them in your life. The adage of less is more holds true in this case since we really do not require a great deal to provide happiness. Once you determine what is important to you, you must strive to live by these principles by infusing and embodying them as your truth.

Make a list of those things in your life which take up your valuable energy and resources but do not deliver the same level of joy, fulfillment and happiness. Do not be persuaded by what you should be doing as since it is a simple choice that brings you closer towards happiness or pulls you further away.

The moment you ask empowering questions and start living the answers, you will be making a statement to the universe declaring the life you wish to lead. Your thoughts, words and actions become your affirmations toward life. So you create meaning to life by first deciding and embarking upon the life that you wish to live. Your statement to the universe is your degree in which you are prepared to work towards your passion and your purpose.

Finally, to give meaning and purpose to your life, choose to live by a set of principles, beliefs and values which are uniquely yours. Do not be swayed or coerced into believing what others believe just because it is the popular thing to do. This will never get you far in life. Some people spend their entire life buying into a concept of what is right for them to find that they had it all wrong after all.

Chapter Summary:

- The power is in your hands. Grow and evolve in order to become a bigger player.

- Simplify life by determining what is most important to you in life? Live these principles and embody them.

- Live your passion and purpose that allows you to create meaning to your life – you are the storyteller, so create a great story.

- Eliminate that which is not conducive to your potential – thoughts, beliefs, people etc.

- Do not wish or hope for things to change without becoming or offering more to life in return.

- When you step up to the plate, life greets you with the equal enthusiasm and more will be given to you each time.

- Define your life, not by what you do, rather by who you ARE.

- What do you stand and live for? What is the essence of your soul? What is your purpose and are you living it to its fullest? Do not allow life to define you.

- Be of service to others – how may I serve and use my talents, skills and genius to create a better situation for others and have fun along the way? Do not wait for someone else to do it first.

- Create a set of principles, beliefs and values to live by. Challenge them and update them as you find new ways.

CHAPTER TWENTY

Living the Lessons

Allow Life to Flow Through You

"Life is a series of natural and spontaneous changes. Don't resist them – that only creates sorrow. Let reality be reality. Let things flow naturally forward in whatever way they like."

Lao-Tzu

We have reached the final chapter in *Navigate Life* and hopefully you will have gained a greater perspective on the essential principles in order to successfully *Navigate Life*. In this final chapter of living the lessons, I encourage you to allow the process of life to flow through you rather than resisting events that show up in your life. When you become the conduit and expression of life by allowing it to flow through you, you are offering less resistance to what is essentially taking place. A great deal of suffering may be attributed to the resistance offered when situations do not go according to plan. Saying *yes* to life and greeting it with passion means that you embrace and envelop every moment, irrespective of whether you believe the moment brings you joy, pain or suffering. There is a greater plan that is unfolding in your life right now and whilst it may seem to the contrary from where you stand, the greater picture suggests that each event and situation taking place in your life has been perfectly orchestrated for your benefit.

We often resist that which we believe is unwarranted and in doing so we attempt to escape the situation by ignoring or denying it. Whatever is happening to you right now is perfect and cannot be made otherwise. The moment you begin to accept this perfection of life, the sooner you will suffer less and enjoy the fulfillment that awaits you. We can choose pain or suffering or we can choose to allow.

My favorite silent mantra is the phrase *I allow*, which I silently repeat when events and situations emerge which my ego labels as unwarranted. By affirming this simple yet powerful statement I am acknowledging anything in my life right now by choosing to not resist the seed of potential of what may become.

There is a difference between yielding to life and succumbing to life. Yield like a tree with supple branches, allowing the wind to blow through it rather than resisting it. When you yield to life, you are allowing the process of life to flow uninterrupted through you. If you resist life, you resist the unfolding of events and circumstances that are necessary to shape your reality. We never really know what life has planned for us, yet underlying all this we hold onto a fear that it might not work as we planned or envisioned and therefore we resist "what is," instead of allowing it. Through yielding you are working with the forces of life by stepping aside and acknowledging that you do not have all the pieces of the puzzle just yet and you are willing to let life show you step by step. We must accept that the creative intelligence cleverly orchestrates the universe and knows what it is doing better than we do.

When I began this journey, I recall the frustration and trepidation cursing through me at the thought of allowing life to know better than me. I would ask myself, *how could a Universe, or force which I cannot see and does not interact with me, know what I want and what is best for me?* But slowly and surely, and with the passage of time, I allowed life to reveal itself through me by first, offering no resistance to what unfolded and then suspending judgment until the sequence of events unfolded.

There is a bigger picture to your life and when you step back from the day to day drama and invite yourself to allow the story to unfold, you begin to live in awe and splendor. The bigger picture to your life centers on the storyline in which you create as part of your narrative. Are you choosing to be the victim within the drama or do you wish to play a more active role in your life by taking responsibility and action for everything that you create and attract into your life circumstances? Far too many people get caught up in the daily dramas of their life and forget about this narrative so inevitably they find themselves attending to smaller situations which are akin to putting out spot fires.

Do you really want to live a life that means putting out spot fires and in doing so forget about the big picture and that is creating the ideal circumstances of your life? To allow life to flow through you means making a decision not to play the victim but rather become the instigator and active conscious creator of your life's destiny. When you are running around putting out spot fires, a sense of helplessness is likely because you are not in a powerful position of creation, rather you are tending to situations which are beyond your control. However, as you become the conscious attractor and creator of every situation and circumstances in your life, you actively take responsibility and ownership for everything that you own and therefore you were not living by someone else's rules.

As you allow the process of life to flow through you uninterrupted and with stout resistance, your life begins to unfold in the most meaningful way. You move into a state of beauty and majesty. There is joy and beauty in life when we open ourselves to being receptive to the magic and wonder it has to offer.

At times in our life we create self-imposed fortresses to protect us and keep us safe. Our mind protects us from people, place and things that have hurt us in the past and so we retreat and build walls and fortresses to keep us safe from future pain, disappointment and hurt. We form limiting beliefs, attitudes and thoughts, which keep us secure and safe. Life is far more than what we imposed upon ourselves.

Break free from your prison by seeking new experiences that challenge you to become more. In doing so, life greets you with the enthusiasm and shows you there is indeed a pot of gold on the other side of the rainbow, but only if you venture out of your comfort zone. Remember, avoid getting tied to the small stuff because in the end, *it is all small stuff.*

There will come a time when you will look back on your life and wonder why you worried about things that really did not matter at the time. The dramas in your life are not the real point of attraction for you and if you allow them to become that, you miss out on what is pure, blissful and joyful to reveal itself through you.

You have all that you need to live a truly amazing and prosperous life, replete with joy, passion, enthusiasm and a deep fulfillment. Life does not have to be monotonous, boring, lifeless and meaningless—there is another way. Yet that other way exists in your mind but requires you to step out of your conventional ways of viewing life. When you subscribe to a certain position about how life should be, you buy into a way of being that corresponds with that belief. It is important to know that is one way of viewing life and does not represent an accurate view of reality. It is subjective to your past. Yet despite all this, all you need to do is flick the switch to activate the wonderful life that awaits you on the other side of your fears, doubts, anxieties and worries. It is possible to become all that you want to be. It is possible that you can find happiness and joy in this lifetime without being tied to conditions. You do not have to surrender your wholeness to claim this aspect of life. You merely need to step into your own power by choosing to reclaim that part of you that you thought was missing, lost or abandoned.

Chapter Summary:

- Become a conduit and expression of life by allowing it to flow through you, instead of knocking heads with life.

- Say "yes" to life more and more and greet it with passion and excitement.

- Whatever is happening to you right now is perfect and cannot be made otherwise. Thinking or believing so creates pain and suffering.

- Pain and suffering are indicators that you have strayed from what is important and what you must attend to now.

- Consent to whatever shows up with little or no resistance by stepping into it, even if that means pain and suffering.

- Every experience and event has the potential to teach you something valuable if you are willing to embrace it. Resistance is futile since life will always win.

- There is a difference between yielding to life and succumbing to life. Yield like a tree with supple branches, allowing the wind to blow through it, rather than resisting it.

- Show up for life and learn to grow through your experiences because that is what your soul has planned for you.

- Learn to embrace the NOW by stepping out of your past or the future. Be present minded orientated and discover the beauty and majesty of riding the blissful wave of life.

- Seek the positive lesson within each experience by refusing to dwell on the negative, despite how dire things may often seem. Seek inner guidance.

- There is a bigger picture to your life. When you step back from the day to day drama and invite yourself to allow the story to unfold; you begin to live in awe and splendor.

- Do not sweat the small stuff because in the end, it is all small stuff.

CHAPTER TWENTY ONE
Conclusion

Your Journey to Freedom Begins

"You are already free. You only have to know and realize this truth."
Sivananda

Congratulations on reaching this far into the book. I trust that the principles and lessons contained within served you well and that you have taken the time to not only understand the concepts on a mental level, but also to embody them on a physical level. In order to make positive changes in our lives we need to create change at a cellular level and continue to practice and rehearse these new changes until such time they become second nature and subconscious. Allow yourself some time to find your ground as you transition from your old ways into the new and exciting way of life.

People often ask me, *Tony, how will I know when I am living these principles in my daily life?* You will know when your previous challenges and problems begin to melt away and you find yourself in a new and exciting place that once was not possible. I recall years ago living a life that was stressful and consumed by things which really did not matter to me in the long term. There came a point when I had to choose between letting go of things which no longer served me, or clutching at situations and problems that was steeped in an emptiness and cycle of unending setbacks. Thankfully, I managed to find my way and after implementing many of these principles into my life, I soon discovered that my previous stressors and challenges no longer had the same effect on me as they did all those years ago.

I noticed that I began to look at problems with a new mind and with a higher state of awareness and consciousness. Inspirational speaker and author Dr Wayne Dyer said, *change the way you look at things and the things you look at change.* Many people attempt to change their external circumstances hoping that all those toxic influences in their lives will miraculously vanish the moment they get rid of them. Unfortunately, life is far more intelligent than we give her credit for as challenges may resurface in order to teach you valuable lessons.

Instead of changing your external environment, *Navigate Life* helps you to readjust to your external world by empowering you with the mental, emotional and spiritual resources to allow you the inner freedom to live the life that you truly deserve. In essence you are either *Navigating Life, Parked* or in a transitory state between the two. There are no mistakes in life and whilst our naive, ego minds likes to believe that there is no master plan, ultimately there is a greater and infinite creative intelligence that governs our entire lives the moment we step into and reclaim our power. Even a so-called "mistake" or what you might call a "disaster" presents itself as an opportunity if framed correctly for both inner and outer growth. There is always a lesson to be gained from each experience in life.

If we get to look close enough, and with an open heart and mind, we can see that upon the threshold of existence lays the foundation of the most magnificent treasure that you will ever know. You are being taking care of within the universe and your needs are always being met. Yet in order to allow yourself the opportunity to step into this magnificent splendor you must let go of all the false and negative lies that we have accumulated in our life. In every situation that presents itself to you, lies the opportunity to advance forward and *Navigate Life* or to remain stagnant and *Parked.* Yet the beauty of the universe is that even whilst you are *Parked* the opportunity to advance is still contained within that very essence of where you stand.

It is for this reason that one of the chapters in the book was deliberately named, *A Quality Life Demands Quality Questions*. The value and quality of questions that you give thought to has the power to impact your life at such a monumental level that it pails into significance against the backdrop of your current problems and challenges.

Many people have reported that since following these principles, areas of their life, which brought them a great deal of discomfort, suddenly becomes so much easier to manage.

The key components to *Navigating Life* are to simplify, simplify, simplify. I cannot stress enough the importance of removing that which is not needed or wanted in your life. Mother Nature does not complicate what it can simplify and since you are an extension of the same energy, it stands to reason that the more you tune yourself to this same creative process, the simpler and easier your life begins to unfold.

I want you to understand that you do not need to suffer and believe that life is about suffering and hardship. There is a lot more to life than you realize. You can leave behind your preconceived ideas and beliefs about how life should unfold. You can choose within any moment to leave behind your suffering and move into are a greater understanding and awareness that you are more than your problems, your regrets and your past mistakes.

As you gain greater mental clarity and move from a *Parked* state to a *Navigating* state, you will be more attuned to an accurate representation of your inner world.

As a conscious creator you to have the power to create your life according to the principles espoused in this book. There is no rush and no deadline for you to follow. Your mind creates these deadlines believing that when you have acquired or achieved a certain goal or wish, you will be fulfilled. That is your ego talking, since your true essence, your spirit is not limited to time nor circumstances. It has its own agenda and can never be hurried along.

Finally, I leave you with the following wisdom which will serve you well along your path to *Navigating Life.*

Honor your path
When you have the answers which resonate with you, you are committed to honoring your path; despite what roadblocks or obstacles show up.

Be well prepared
Preparation not only means being physically prepared, it also includes mental and emotional preparedness. Knowing that life presents us with ebbs and flows allows you to understand that things will not always go according to your plan. Nonetheless, remain receptive to the cycle of life and in doing so work with the forces of life rather than opposing them. Trust that you are being supported in your endeavors when you honor your path. If you venture outside of your jurisdiction, the universe will advise you in no uncertain terms that it is time to regain your focus.

Remain vigilant
Some of the toughest terrain in the world lay waiting in the recesses of your mind. When you overcome these obstacles, your journey takes on new meaning. Remaining vigilant reminds you to stay committed despite the difficult times ahead. Vigilance is a state of being. It is a way of asserting ones mental state, despite the external conditions. You remain poised and receptive that your journey will be fulfilled.

The principles outlined operate in harmony when applied. You cannot have one without the other. Reflect on this for a moment— your reward far exceeds anything that life will throw at you. Use these principles as foundations to successfully navigate your way toward the life of your dreams. Make a commitment that you will remain on the path no matter what challenges you face. Have faith that you will be shown the path ahead as you approach the crossroads of life. The bridge serves as a connection between the past and the future. Be bold and daring! Cross each bridge and in doing so, pave the way ahead to a magical and prosperous life.

There are no mistakes!

Navigation Questionnaire

Tick the boxes in the columns below which you MOST identify with, to discover if you are NAVIGATING life or PARKED. Your answers will assist you making informed decisions to move forward in life.

Life View

PARKED	NAVIGATING
☐ Everything feels like a chore	☐ Your actions arise from inspiration
☐ There is no 'life' in your day to day tasks	☐ Every day is gift and a blessing
☐ You often see everything as a challenge instead of an opportunity	☐ Your actions arise from purpose
☐ You often believe you have no choice in life	☐ You transcend all limitations
☐ Life happens to you, not through you	☐ Doors begin to open

Life View

PARKED	NAVIGATING
☐ You may complain and find fault in the smallest details	☐ Everything is easy and effortless
☐ Stress is now chronic. You gravitate toward drinking at night in order to relax and sleeping pills to help you sleep.	☐ You have a well-defined physique with the right balance of muscle to fat.
☐ You often feel disconnected from others	☐ You find joy and meaning in everything you do
☐ There is little sense of purpose in your life and work	☐ Your energy is high, since you're inspired
☐ You may feel life owes you something	☐ You see opportunities in every action and interaction
☐ You live in a state of panic and continual worry i.e. money, health, relationships	☐ Happiness is the way
☐ You feel unfulfilled	☐ Your true nature evolves and shines for others to see
☐ You feel something is missing; though you don't know what	☐ You can't wait to get up in the morning
☐ You feel bored with life	☐ You see beauty in the smallest detail
☐ You're uninterested in world & local issues	☐ You're rarely stressed
☐ You feel as though you demand more on others resources	☐ There is a deep fountain of joy and peacefulness which emanates from within

Life View

PARKED	NAVIGATING
☐ You may feel unexplained anxiety and fear at times	☐ You're grounded by living in the present moment
☐ There is never enough time in your day	☐ You're oblivious to time when you work or play
☐ You're stressed at work. It feels as though everything is a challenge	☐ You achieve more by doing less
☐ Problems are just annoying things which get in the way	☐ You see the synchronicity and lessons in every experience
TOTAL SCORE:	TOTAL SCORE:

Relationships

PARKED	NAVIGATING
☐ You may feel disengaged from certain relationships	☐ You have fulfilling, stable relationships with loved ones, friends and family
☐ You feel as though loved ones and friends just don't 'understand' you	☐ You see the beauty of relationships as growth and learning
☐ You're often disconnected from others, spending time alone perhaps	☐ You attend to relationships in a nurturing and caring manner
☐ You're frustrated in relationships. Looking for a way out	☐ You use relationships to grow and evolve as a person

Relationships

PARKED	NAVIGATING
☐ The smallest things in others may set you off at times	☐ You love being in the company of friends, family and colleagues often

TOTAL SCORE: TOTAL SCORE:

Health & Wellbeing

PARKED	NAVIGATING
☐ You may neglect your health and your body at times	☐ You radiate health, wellness and vitality
☐ You might drink often seeking comfort in alcohol to unwind and relax	☐ You thrive on moving your body through exercise
☐ You often have low energy levels; suffering from tiredness and fatigue	☐ You respect and value your body as a vehicle for experiencing life
☐ You may rely on external stimulants to keep you going i.e. coffee, sugar, alcohol	☐ You nourish your body with exercise, sleep and sound nutrition
☐ You may suffer from insomnia or poor sleep	☐ Your mind is your ally as is your body
☐ You suffer digestive related symptoms at most of the time i.e. bloating, distension, wind, cramps, discomfort	☐ You radiate a sense of aliveness and unbound energy. You're seldom fatigued

Health & Wellbeing

PARKED	NAVIGATING
☐ You shy away from most forms of exercise	☐ You perform some form of Eastern health ritual i.e. yoga, meditation, qi gong, tai chi
☐ You may feel disconnected from your body. It's like a machine which serves you	☐ Your energy comes from nourishing every living cell from within your body

TOTAL SCORE: TOTAL SCORE:

Attitudes, Thoughts & Beliefs

PARKED	NAVIGATING
☐ You may experience scattered thoughts at times, unable to break the cycle	☐ You're a conscious creator of your life and future
☐ You feel trapped in your current circumstances	☐ Failure is just another way to get 'get it right'
☐ You can't wait to go on holidays to take a break from work	☐ You don't strive or resist life. Life unfolds through you
☐ You find yourself complaining about lack of money, support, opportunities etc.	☐ There's no need to compete with others
☐ You may be cynical, believing the worst in situations as distinct from the best outcome	☐ You're in alignment with your thoughts and emotions. They serve you.

Attitudes, Thoughts & Beliefs

PARKED	NAVIGATING
☐ You find it a challenge to see two sides to a situation	☐ You're open and receptive to the flow of information and ideas
☐ You're apathetic to challenges and changes in your life, choosing things to remain as they are	☐ You let go of things which no longer serve you i.e. things, people, places, ideas and emotions
☐ You may have a stubborn streak; not willing to embrace alternative views	☐ You're not a victim to your thoughts i.e. cause & effect
☐ You may be restless and often frustrated	☐ You remain positive with your attitudes & beliefs toward life
TOTAL SCORE:	TOTAL SCORE:

Emotions

PARKED	NAVIGATING
☐ You find it difficult to show your emotions at times, seeing this as a noticeable weakness perhaps	☐ You're in alignment with your thoughts and emotions. They serve you well
☐ You're not attuned to your emotional constitution	☐ You're emotionally stable. Experiencing neither high or low bouts
☐ You may not understand your emotions and tend to stuff things under the carpet	☐ Your outer world does not affect inner world. You remain poised and often unaffected by drama
☐ Your emotions may fluctuate from highs and lows	☐ You regard your 'emotional intelligence' as high

Emotions

PARKED	NAVIGATING
☐ You may react to external stimuli; allowing things outside of you to affect you emotionally	☐ You don't ruminate and dwell on problems, allowing them to affect you emotionally

TOTAL SCORE: TOTAL SCORE:

Career & Business

PARKED	NAVIGATING
☐ You may feel disengaged from your work and relationships	☐ Your purpose is your career. It is your joy and passion
☐ You feel unfulfilled in your job and/or career	☐ Your career is a calling and not just a means of earning a living or a wage. It provides you a deep sense of satisfaction.
☐ There may be little sense of purpose in your work	☐ Work is an opportunity to express your true talent and genius
☐ You work in a job to get paid a salary and remain content with delivering as much as you need to	☐ You work hard, but don't call it work. It feel as though you're caught up in play; remaining oblivious to time

TOTAL SCORE: TOTAL SCORE:

Money & Finance

PARKED	NAVIGATING
☐ You may complain about having lack of money at times	☐ You're not concerned with the flow of money into your life
☐ You hold limiting beliefs around money i.e. 'money doesn't grow on trees'	☐ Money flows into your life with ease and perfection
☐ You may think in terms of scarcity or lack. There is not enough to go around	☐ You continually think in terms of abundance and prosperity. You have a positive relationship with money
☐ You find yourself continually in debt or owing money and never 'getting ahead'	☐ You give money away – tithing, charity etc.
☐ Money is hard to come by. You find yourself working hard to make money and its 'hard to come by, easy to go'	☐ You allow money to flow through you as a channel. You neither hoard or squander money
☐ You may often find that money issues impose upon your quality of life	☐ You appreciate the qualities of money, not as something to worship, rather as a means to live a fulfilling life
TOTAL SCORE:	TOTAL SCORE:

Self Awareness & Spirituality

PARKED	NAVIGATING
☐ You may be apprehensive and skeptical about that which you cannot see	☐ You practice some form of spiritual service regularly

Self Awareness & Spirituality

PARKED	NAVIGATING
☐ You feel that you need to 'see' evidence before believing in something	☐ You're connected to a higher source of intelligence
☐ You find is challenging sitting in silence to meditate as it means being alone with your thoughts	☐ You have a worldly connection to others. You think universally and act local
☐ You may feel a sense of emptiness and unfulfilled within	☐ You meditate often and enjoy being in nature
☐ Something is missing or longing in your life, yet you don't know what it is	☐ You believe in an infinite intelligence which created you and the universe
☐ You may be critical of others at times and not making time to hear other people's view	☐ You believe without seeing
☐ You're find yourself judgmental at times	☐ You thrive on being in your own company. It's an opportunity to go within

TOTAL SCORE:

TOTAL SCORE:

Overall Score Parked:

Overall Score Navigating:

Other Great Titles by Heart Space Publications

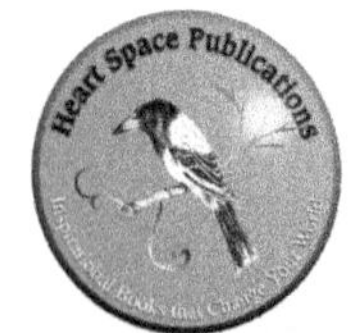

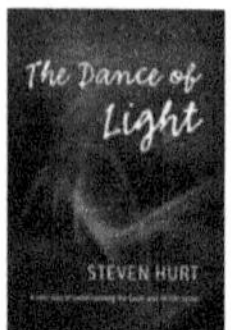

Dance of Light: a new way of understanding the Earth and all life forms

All is One : an extra ordinary book that teaches difficult concepts in a simple way!

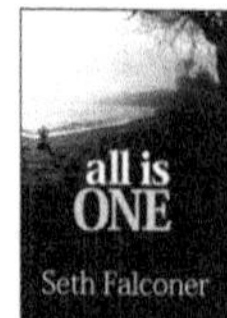

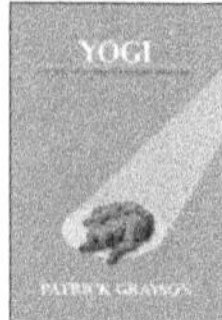

Yogi, the Tails and Teachings of a Suburban Alpha Doggy: a delightful read illustrating the wisdom and humour that animals bring to our lives

Second Chance, Regain your Health with Tissue Salts: this book will help the full spectrum of users, from concerned parents, experienced pharmacists and health care workers

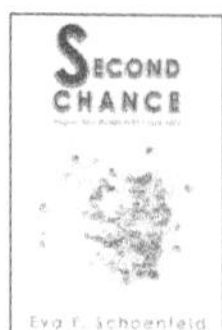

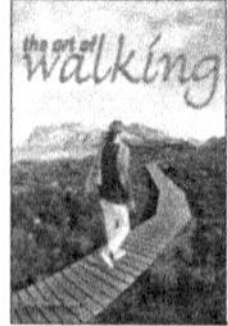

The Art of Walking: a treasure trove of knowledge, practical guidance and inspiration in lyrical prose

Know Thyself: a workbook that can become a lifeline for alife that works

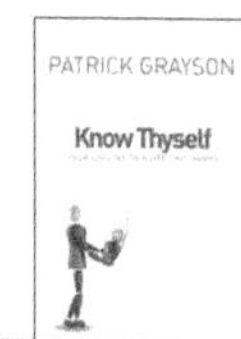

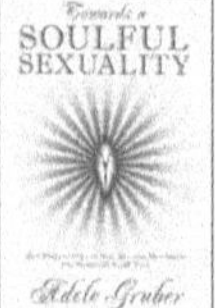

Towards a Soulful Sexuality: an intelligent, thought provoking and candid new perspective of sex, age and menopause for all women.

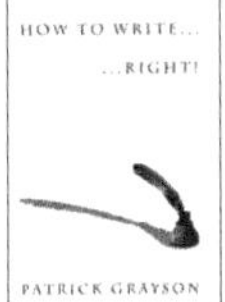

How to Write - Right!: with this book you will become the writer you have always wanted to be

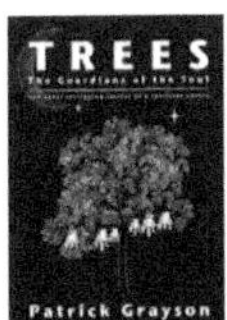

Trees, the Guardian of the Soul: a book of short stories that imparts the wisdom of the ages, appealing to all age groups

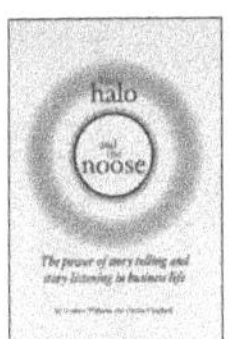

The Halo and the Noose: a great piece of work which stimulates one to look at life differently

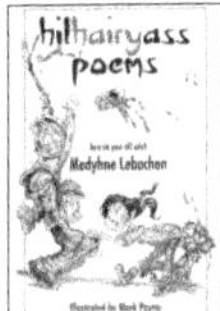

Hillhairyass Poems: poems and illustrations created to entertain and support young adults

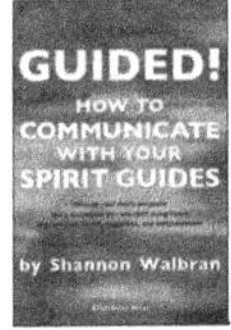

Guided! How to Communicate with your Spirit Guides: Discover your soul's purpose and learn techniques to communicate with your spirit guides

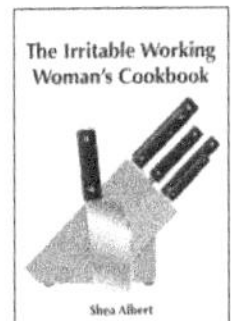

The Irritable Woman's Cookbook: "cooking is like sex; you have to be in the mood", says the humorous author of this Jewish cookbook

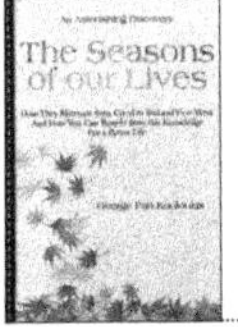

The Seasons of Our Lives: George Kouloukis shows that the alternating trends of our lives - going from good to bad and vice versa, are according to specific patterns.

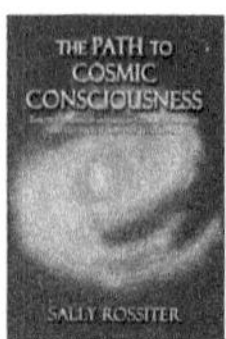

The Path of Cosmic Consciousness: journey through initiation to enlightenment in the sacred Andean tradition

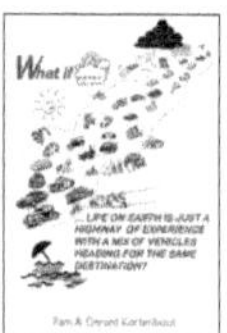

What if: an encounter of simple truth about life and spirituality

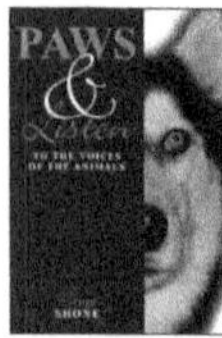

Paws and Listen to the Voices of the Animals: Read this book, then open your heart, free your mind and listen to the ancient wisdom of the animals that you love.

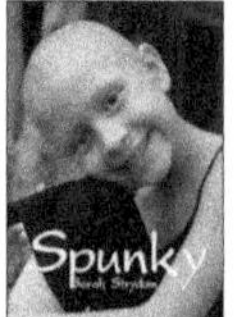

Spunky: Join me on my journey of becoming a cancer survivor, and against all odds a provincial badminton player.

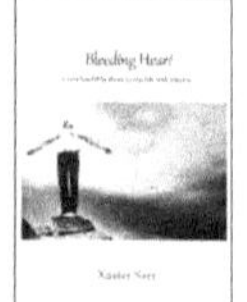

Bleeding Heart: Bleeding Heart is a timeless fable about living life with passion. It will bring joy to your soul as you turn the pages ever faster.

Heart Space Publications

Australia: +61 450 260 348

South Africa: +27 11 431 1274

pat@heartspacebooks.com

www.heartspacebooks.com